in search of charm

Dictionary definition of Charm *Enchantment in the eyes of others*

James Barrie's definition of Charm *A sort of bloom on a woman*

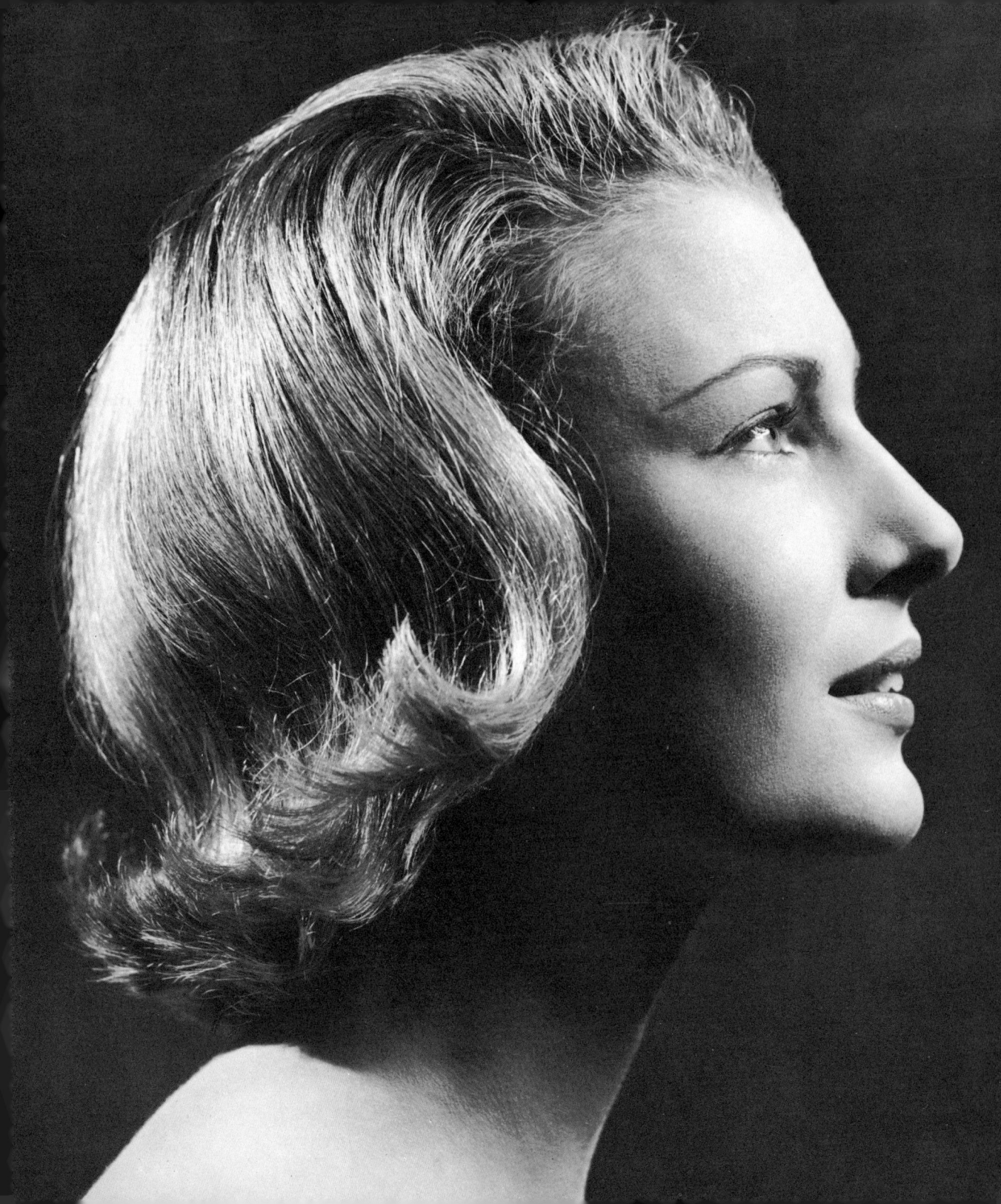

in search of charm

MARY YOUNG

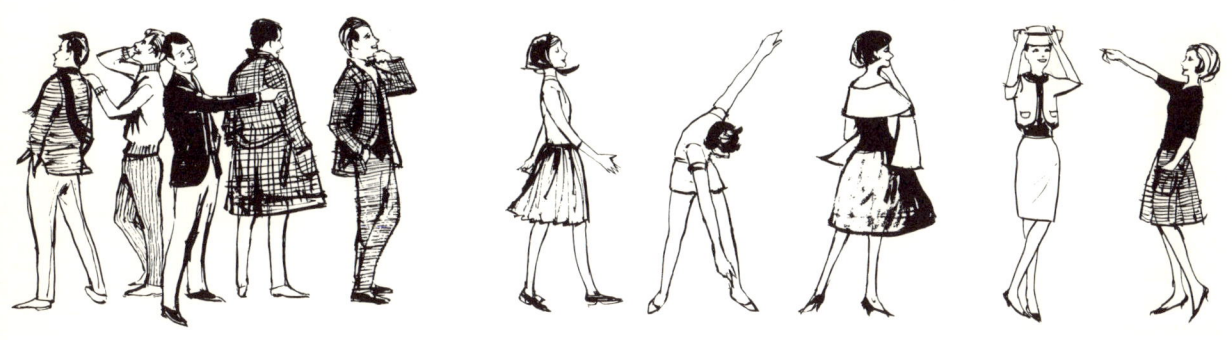

The World Publishing Company

The book is designed and illustrated by the Peter Hatch Partnership Ltd
Designer: Richard Daynes M S I A
Drawings by Donald Gott

Photographs by Nancy Sandys Walker F B I P and Dennis Hughes-Gilbey
Our thanks are due to British Lion Films Ltd for permission
to reproduce a photograph of Cyd Charisse; and to Twentieth
Century-Fox Film Company Ltd for a photograph of Sophia Loren

First printed 1962
Published by Brockhampton Press Ltd, Market Place, Leicester
Text copyright © 1962 by Mary Young
Illustrations copyright © 1962 by Peter Hatch Partnership Ltd
First United States Printing 1965
Copyright © 1965 by Mary Young and Peter Hatch Partnership Ltd
Published by The World Publishing Company
2231 West 110th Street
Cleveland 2, Ohio
Library of Congress Catalog Card Number: 65-15119

	introduction	6	
1	**where do I start?**	8	*A balanced personal appraisal*
2	**first things first**	13	*Facial expression — posture*
3	**deportment**	19	*Walking — standing — sitting — mannerisms*
4	**figure**	27	
5	**makeup**	39	
6	**dress**	46	
7	**grooming**	57	*Freshness — perfume — care of the body — hair*
8	**personality**	68	*Definition — guidance — self-reliance — poise*
9	**voice and laughter**	72	
10	**etiquette and behavior**	75	*An evening out with your boy friend — restaurant — eating points — introductions — smoking*
11	**interviews**	89	*Outfit and appearance — questions to expect*
12	**first job**	93	*First days — meeting other employees — standard of behavior — personal equipment — wolves*
13	**an apartment of your own**	96	*Points for easy running — organization — entertaining*
14	**a few points to round off the whole**	100	
	supplement	103	*Wearing clothes like a model*

introduction

During the long years I have devoted to training models or advising girls and women on what is generally called charm, but which I call self-improvement, I have never for a moment considered that this was a subject worth expounding in a book. I always feel that the essence of my teaching (and any benefits my pupils may have derived from it) is in the human touch, the personal approach and the individual attention. No one, therefore, was more surprised than myself when, following an article in the *Observer* and a television appearance, I was approached to write a book on the things I teach.

Not being a professional writer, I sat down with considerable reluctance to accomplish this task and, in giving it to my publisher, I felt a certain trepidation at the thought that so many of the things I would like to explain personally, or to demonstrate, might be misunderstood by readers who are of necessity confined to the printed word. This is not a subject which is easy to condense into a teach-yourself form.

Although I have often considered myself to be something of a jack-of-all-trades, my various interests, studies and experiences have somehow welded themselves into the whole that is necessary for Fashion Model Training and Charm Courses. I now find it fascinating when I am asked to adapt this whole for classes labeled "Poise, Dress and Personality" (for London County Council), for courses for factories, stores and offices, down to single lectures for such groups as the Soroptimists. As a matter of fact, since I run my own Model Agency as well as organizing the training and lecturing activities, I am thankful for my years in a very busy office and for experience with two Ministries.

However, it was my years as a teacher and exponent of Natural Movement Dancing that led me into the fashion world. I discovered to my delight that the grace of movement, control of gesture, command of expression, as well as the spontaneity inherent in this type of dancing (which originated with Isadora Duncan) were ideal for training the model. When I was developing the overall training, I came more and more to the conclusion that this was what every young woman wants, something to give her poise, a dress sense and confidence in herself, and thus was born my enthusiasm for taking my activities into wider fields, one of which is this book.

It is this poise, dress sense and confidence that you will see at a Fashion Parade, or in a lovely film star. Maybe you have in your mind a picture of the beautiful, poised young woman you would like to be yourself.

This is the point of this book—how to set about becoming that poised, enchanting young woman. Not to become like some top model whom you admire! But to become a young woman with your own particular brand of charm simply because you have allowed your individuality and inherent abilities to develop and bloom, and because at the same time you have worked hard to make the very best of your appearance.

"Ladies," said Mr. Samuel Goldwyn, the famous Hollywood producer, "if you want to be devastating, use all the arts of sophistication, but remain *demure*."

Now the phrase "the arts of sophistication" conjures up good grooming, elegant dressing, beauty culture in all its aspects, poise and grace of movement, good speech and a developed personality; "demure" suggests that tenderness, sweetness and serenity without which no woman can be truly beautiful. And if this book tends to dwell on the arts of sophistication, it is because I can't stress too strongly that I feel the young woman of today should be that well-balanced person suggested by a wise Mr. Goldwyn.

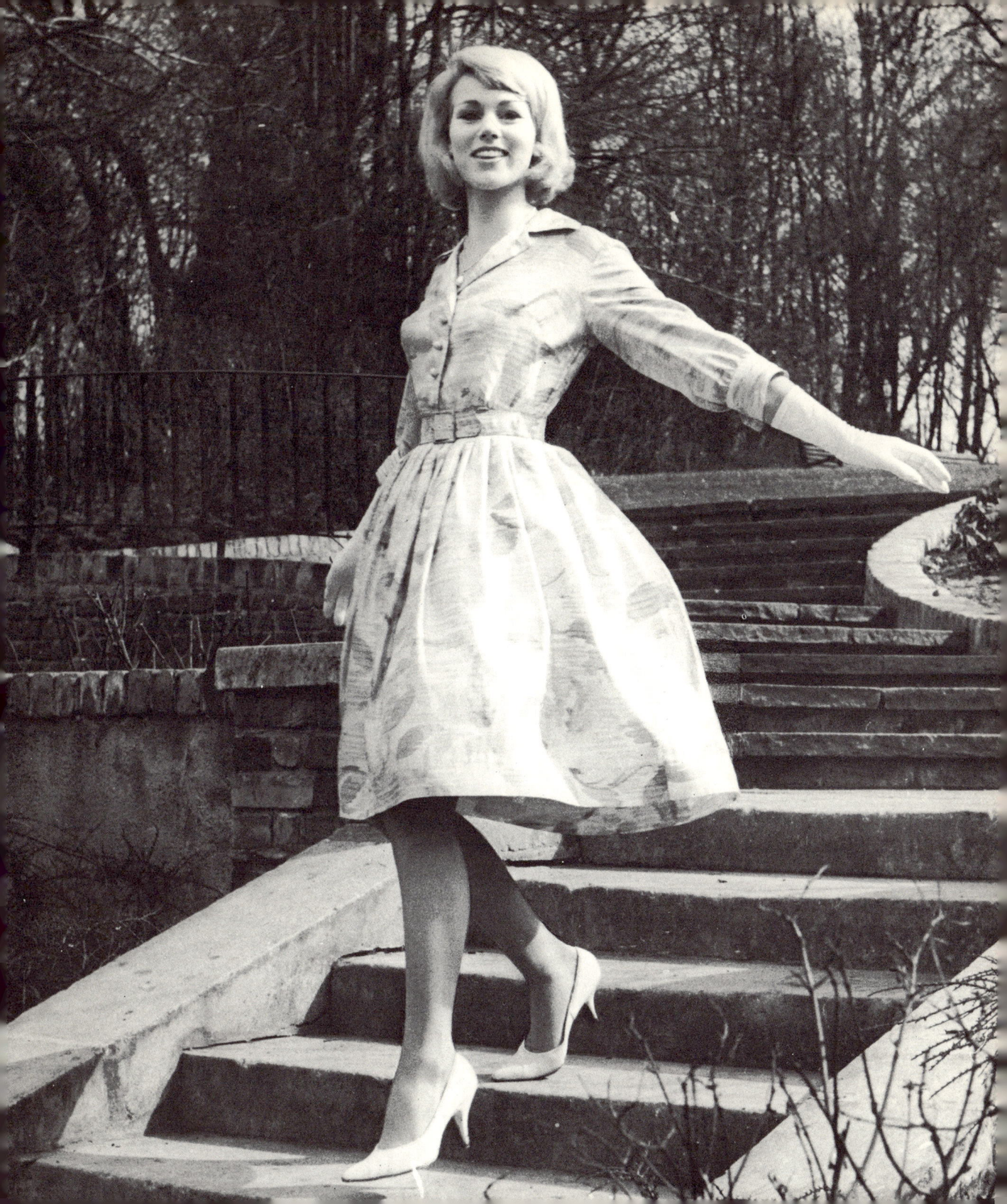

1 where do I start?

This chapter could just as easily be labeled *where do I stop?* There are many ordinary and everyday activities which by being overdone, done in the wrong way, or, in some cases, done at all, may be spoiling your looks, figure or grooming. Perhaps you are a sports girl and have set your heart upon winning medals and cups, becoming a champion something or other, or even swimming the Channel. There is nothing wrong with this as long as you are sure that everything is well balanced by the feminine things of life.

muscles

The famous prima ballerinas we all admire *do not* have oversize muscles and yet—in order to keep at the top of their profession—they continually keep in training. They are able to keep slim, lithe limbs by following accepted methods of releasing and relaxing muscles that have been strenuously used. Leave it to the men to develop sheer size of muscle and glory in it. My ideal girl has a slim, strong body with firm contours and not a muscle in sight.

swimming

If you're mad about swimming, take a look at your upper arm and the top part of the body to see whether there is any overdevelopment. Everyone ought to be able to swim. Moreover, swimming is a particularly fine activity which combines development of muscle, breathing capacity, and grace of movement. But unless that championship means more to you than anything else, then indulge only in moderation, and after all swimming sessions be sure to shake out and generally flex the muscles that have been most in use.

riding

If you are keen on riding, then watch for possible overdevelopment of the upper thigh muscles. When you come to wear your first straight skirt or dress, you are going to be heartbroken if you find that your thighs measure more than your hips. A thigh bulge is very difficult to get rid of; so beware, and ride only in moderation, and, again, flex and shake out, the muscles that have been used most.

bicycling

If you are riding a bicycle, don't indulge in the competition of racing when going up hills. Ignore the prowess of your best friend, or the jeers of your brother and *his* friends, and just get off with great dignity and walk. Otherwise you may be subjecting your whole body to quite unnecessary strain.

hockey

If you play hockey and get your hands bruised or scratched over and over again—usually in the same place—then wear protective gloves or at least fingerguards where your fingers are most vulnerable. The damage done to hands by continual knocks on the same spot can be permanent.

tennis

To be able to play tennis is almost a social must, but if you are an enthusiast you may find you are overdeveloping the muscles of your playing arm. If so, between sets, get the habit of shaking out and flexing the arm that is doing all the work.

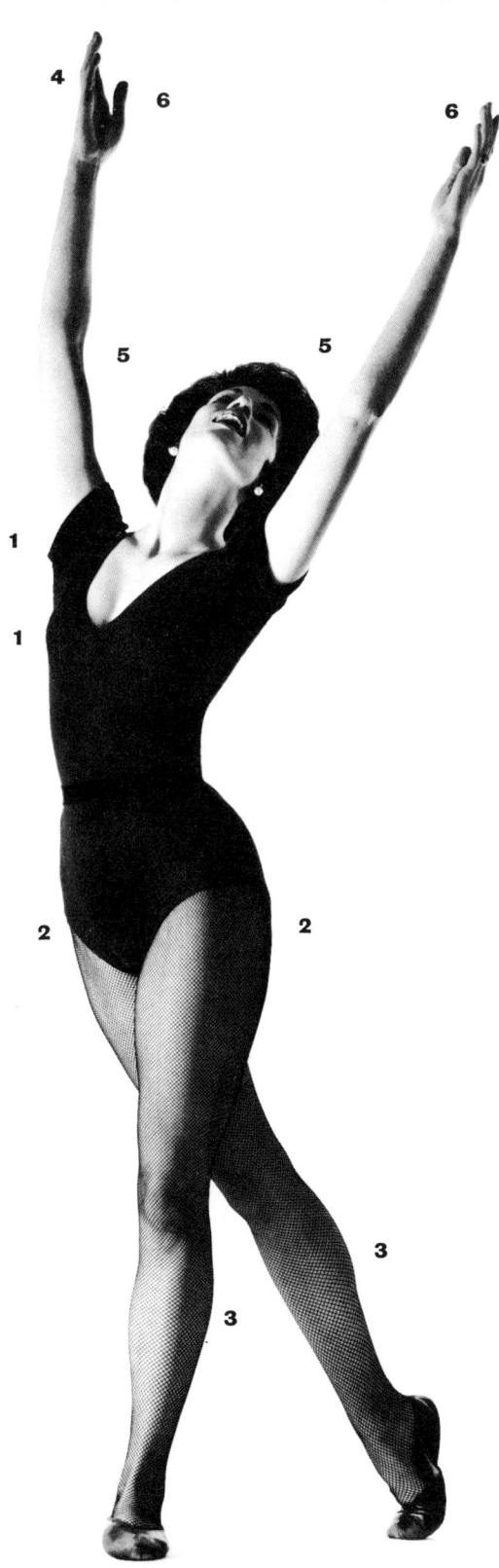

sports that affect your body

1 *swimming*
2 *riding*
3 *bicycling*
4 *hockey*
5 *tennis*
6 *rowing*

rowing

When my brother (rampageous type) and I were fifteen and fourteen we developed a passion for rowing. We spent all our pocket money hiring boats (quite unknown to our parents, and I've often wondered since that the boatkeepers weren't worried about us). Often rowing miles against a strong current, I was always determined to keep up with my brother, and even to this day I have hardish patches in the palms of my hands where time and time again I got blisters from overdoing the rowing.

frowns and lines

Do you frown, scowl, pull down your mouth, or create lines on your forehead? If so, it's quite definitely "stop" to all of these, because the lines created in this way can be aging, ugly, and definitely unattractive. For the moment, just do your best to keep your face serene and happy-looking. If you find this difficult, then rest assured that we shall go more deeply into this further on.

feet

Do you know that tight, ill-fitting, uncomfortable shoes or neglected feet can actually make you feel irritable and bad-tempered—not to mention the resulting frowns and scowls? If you wear shoes that are uncomfortable you will ruin the appearance of your feet and it really is a pity to go through life ashamed of them. Before buying new shoes, ask yourself, "Which means more to me, the appearance of my *footwear* or the appearance of my *feet?*"

spotty, muddy complexion

For this confidence-stealing complaint practically every skin specialist would advise giving up chocolates, sweets, pastry, fried foods and eating more salads, fruits, and green vegetables. If, in addition to having a poor complexion you are overweight—then there's a still further reason for laying off the fattening foods.

personal balanced appraisal

Finally, *stop* bemoaning the fact that you're not like your favorite film star. We all tend to dislike our own looks—particularly, if I may say so, our own noses. We tend to look at a friend's nose and say, "Now, if only I had a nose like yours...", while she is saying to us, "But your nose is wonderful, it's just what I would choose..." After all, you can never be anyone but yourself, and the sooner you reach a personal, balanced appraisal of yourself the better. It is a pity to wait until you are forty or fifty before appreciating your own inherent good points and doing something about your difficulties. Since coming of age is a milestone in life, decide now that you will look forward to twenty-one as the age when you will have reached an understanding of the poise, charm, elegance, and dress sense that you feel is desirable for your particular life. Then, with all the trials and errors behind you, you will be able to go forward into your twenties with the utmost self-confidence, serenity and with a lasting sense of well-being.

The first thing to do in order to reach a balanced, personal appraisal is to put down on paper your bad, or difficult points *and* your good points. It is as important to realize the qualities that are right or attractive as to criticize faults and shortcomings. All too often I have had a student so obsessed with some bad point that she made herself miserable over the situation, thus entirely overlooking her many good points, of which she was completely unaware. Accept and be thankful for all the good points.

So-called BAD points

I can imagine that when putting down your bad points, you may well include items which tend to bother you, but which may be assets when viewed from a different angle.

a large mouth

Sophia Loren's mouth has often been described as big and ugly, but try to imagine her face with just a normal-

1

Points which you may or may not be aware of, but which will certainly be obvious to the onlooker

Possible GOOD points	**Possible BAD points**
A friendly expression	*A bored or unapproachable look*
A look of reliability	*A flighty look*
A lovely smile	*A too solemn or serious look*
Natural confidence	*Self-consciousness*
An arresting personality	*An uninteresting personality*
A calm, serene, or relaxed manner	*A restless, fidgety or tense manner*
Always punctual	*Late for everything*
Attractive voice and laughter	*A voice or laugh with which "one couldn't live" (or worse, giggles)*
A general all-over neatness	*Untidiness*
Dress sense	*No dress sense*

2

Points for which nature or the way you live may be responsible

A lovely face	*A plain face*
Good bodily proportions	*Difficult figure*
Good posture	*Slack, drooping posture*
Attractive natural coloring	*Uninteresting natural coloring*
Good skin	*Poor skin*
Good hair and hairline	*Unmanageable hair and difficult hairline*
Well-shaped feet and ankles	*Big feet, thick ankles*
Good hands and well-shaped nails	*Large hands, poor nails*

3

Points which you will know yourself

Budget-minded	*Spendthrift*
Good planner	*Nothing ever planned ahead*
A constructive attitude to life generally, particularly to difficulties	*No design for living, a worrier, a drifter*

As a matter of fact you will find that an appraisal on these lines is very searching, so much so that even if you read no further, it would have a remarkable salutary effect upon you.

sized mouth, and you will see that she would then begin to look like many another good-looking film star, and she would have lost a large slice of her individual appearance. Many lovely actresses have large mouths.

a broad jaw line

Consider the far from classical beauty of Grace Kelly's face. But the broad jaw line and the firmly rounded lower cheek are distinctly part of her individual charm.

a long face

A long face isn't necessarily something to disguise at all costs. The length may be its special charm. A Frenchwoman would probably do everything she knew to make her long face look even longer—accepting the length as an asset and knowing that it would be deadly if we all tried to make our faces conform to a pattern.

blushing

If you blush, most people will consider it charming and even becoming, though this may not be much comfort.

the very tall girl

Stop to consider for a moment *why* the world of fashion has invariably sought the tall young woman for its salons, showrooms, and shops, and for modeling. The reason is that height *of itself* seems to give a certain presence to its owner—something which the shorter woman can never have. When height is combined with poise and elegance, the effect is terrific. The tall girl who forever wears flat heels, flat hair styles, throws her head forward, stoops, or generally tries to telescope her body in some way in an effort to make it appear less tall, is probably *ruining* her appearance and posture. I would recommend that the very tall girl wear shoes and hair styles that really suit her, even if they add to her height, and that she move with great dignity, as though she is trying to appear even taller. Only thus can she manage her height as it deserves. People certainly can't miss seeing the tall girl—and she should make certain that in the same breath in which they comment upon her height, they also add, ". . . but, how beautifully she managed it".

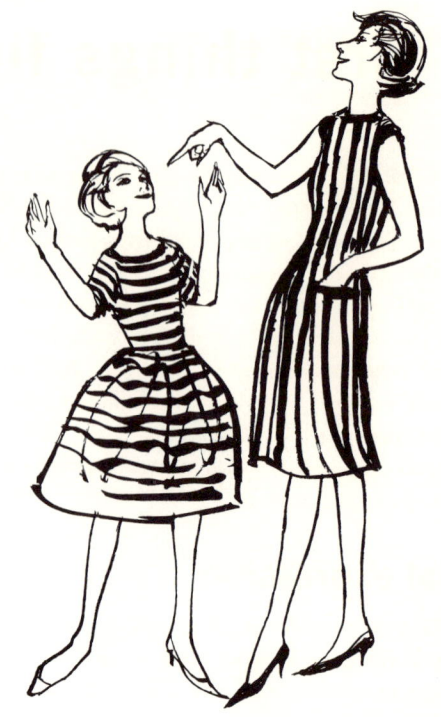

But you needn't emphasize height or shortness . . .

the short girl

Probably the greatest asset of the short girl is that she makes men feel protective. Very well—let her accept any extra consideration or courtesies that may come her way. And let her learn to think of herself as neat and trim, and, above all, petite—a truly delightful word.

However, as we go along you will find that there is probably a very great deal that can be done about most of your points which are really bad. Some of them can be cured, and some of them can be minimized or disguised. And if you follow all the counsels of perfection contained in this book, you can become so enchanting that your few remaining bad points will hardly be noticed—or they just won't matter any more.

2 first things first *facial expression and posture*

Even in one brief, momentary glance, facial expression and posture are taken in by the eye of the beholder whether consciously or unconsciously looked for. They cannot be missed. Moreover, character, health, state of being, self-confidence or otherwise, and the sort of person you are tend to be etched into the look on your face and into the carriage of the body. And if you are observant yourself, you may have noticed how many girls you pass in the street seem to be ruining their appearance unnecessarily by an unattractive expression or by a drooping posture.

Facial expression

Something to console us all is that the face that looks back at us from the looking glass is hardly ever the face that looks at others. When we look in the looking glass we tend to give ourselves a cold, hard stare—an empty scrutiny that seems reserved for this moment alone. The moment we turn to others, our face is transformed by the quality of the look, word, or smile, and the onlooker sees the complete merging of the physical looks and the personality. However, we must face the fact that the unpleasant, uncharitable or unfriendly thought, look, or word will hardly make us appear more attractive, and that frowning, looking harassed or sorry for ourselves drains away our beauty and seems to add years to our appearance. On the other hand, tenderness, compassion, affection, and friendliness will weave their own magic into the normal contours of the face. How many times have I seen a basically plain, rather tired business-girl (even without makeup) looking nevertheless for the time being quite beautiful *because* her joy at being with the young man with whom she is in love is lighting her whole face.

In due course, I am sure you will develop your own mental mirror, but meanwhile, here are a number of moments in life when a special effort is needed to maintain a serene expression.

In biting winds how can you look attractive with a screwed-up face which seems to be saying: "I just can't bear it." Try relaxing your face to the wind, thinking "wonderful cold wind" and pretending you are thoroughly enjoying it. Everyone passing will be taking a second look at your radiant expression.

In the heat how can you look attractive if you are visibly wilting? Try holding up your face as though you're blissfully reveling in sunshine and warmth. Everyone around will be asking you how you keep so cool.

During hard concentration at work or play how can you look attractive if you spend hours and hours with a frown, lines on your forehead, or a tight mouth? Keep a serene face whatever the pressure.

When traveling how can you look attractive or arrive at your destination cool, calm, and collected if you're working yourself into a nervous tension at every little delay? Once on your vehicle, relax in your seat; even close your eyes.

Looking angry, irritated or impatient if you have any doubts about what these emotions do to your face, just confirm your worst suspicions by making for the nearest looking glass. Your mental mirror will serve forever afterwards. Life will be much happier for you and you will be much easier to live with if you train yourself to be understanding, calm, patient, and sweet *whatever happens.*

Boredom this will inevitably be written all over your

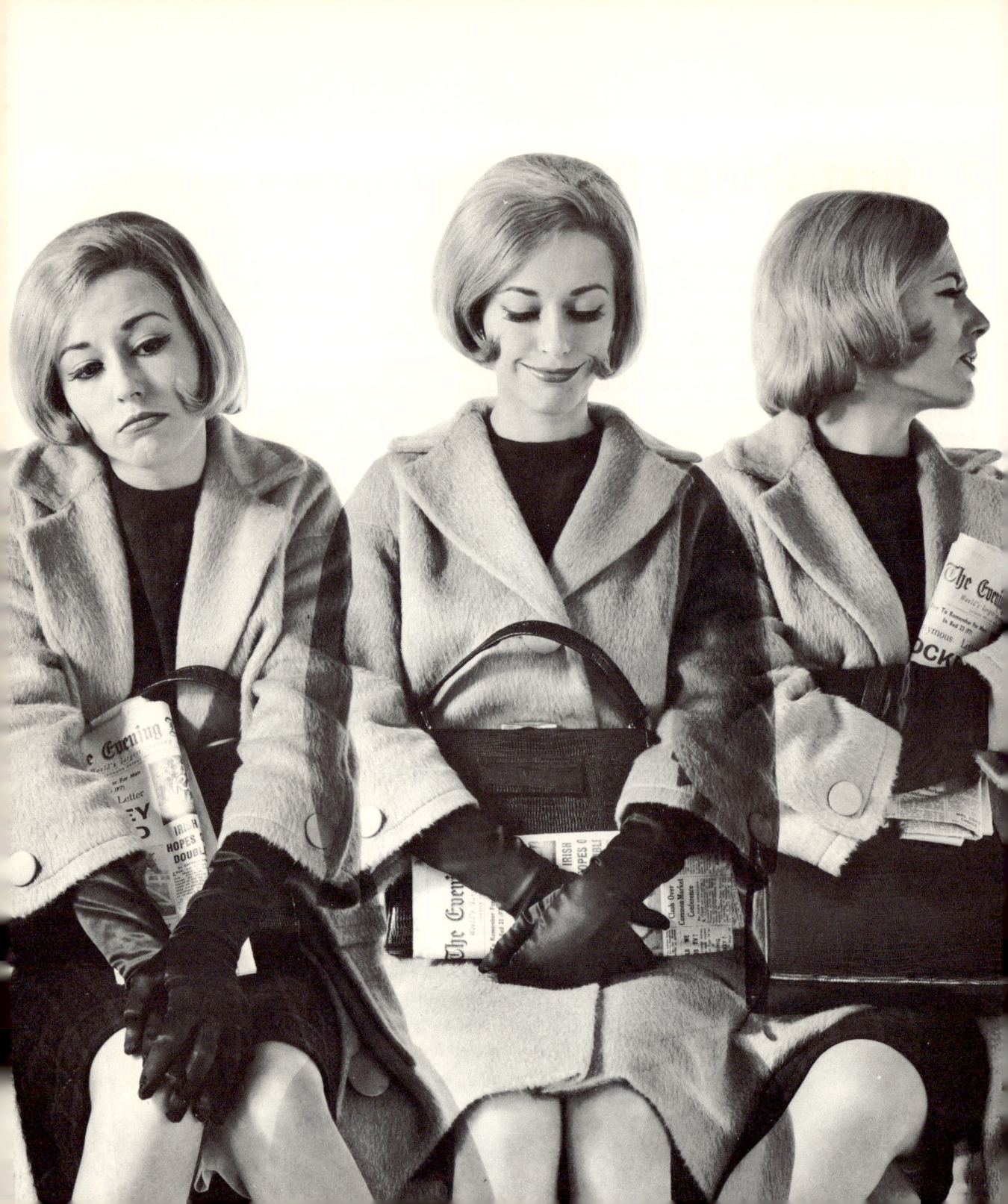

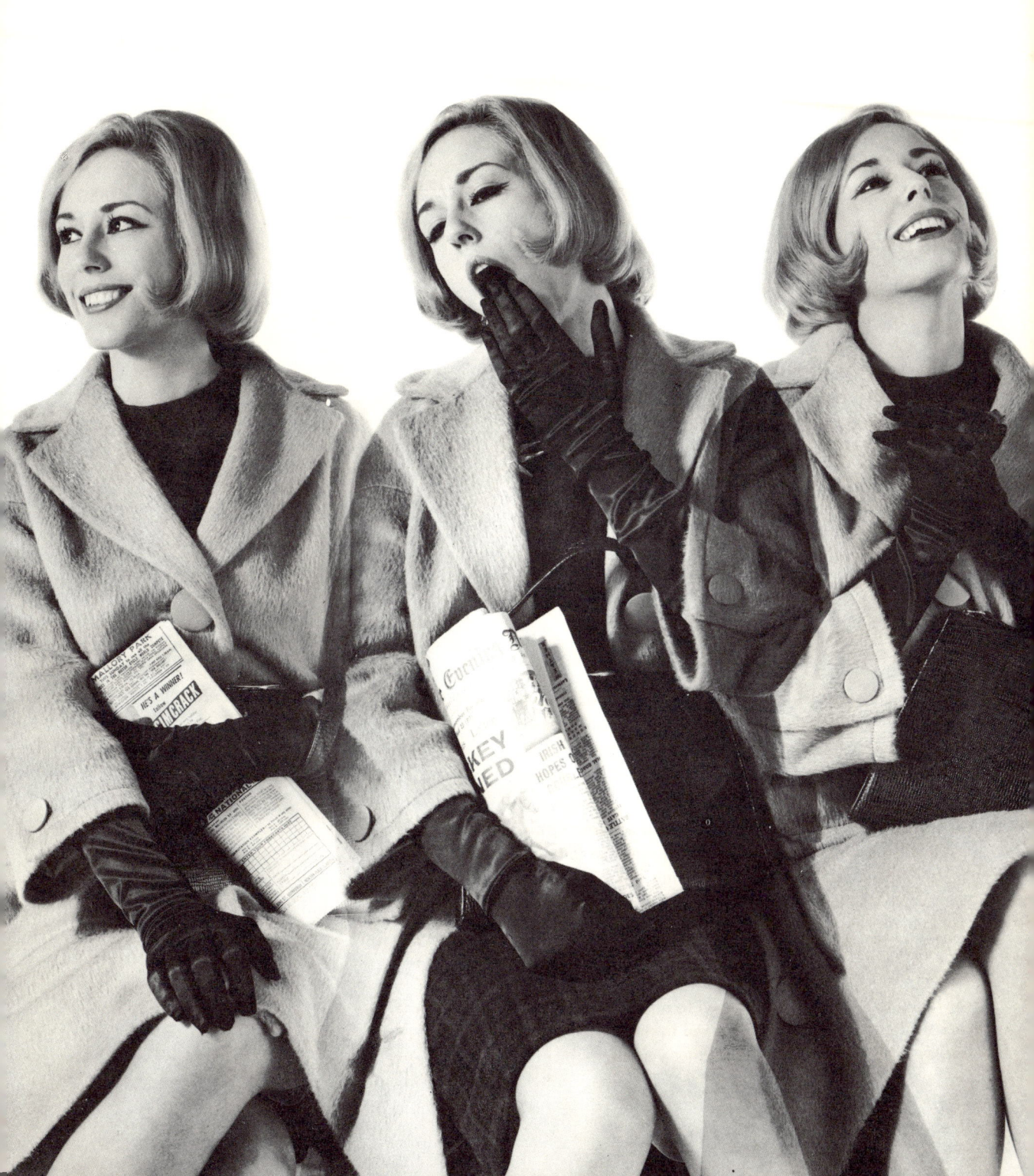

face. Ask yourself what is wrong with you when the world is chock-full of interest or need in all directions. Try tuning in to everything and everybody around you. Boredom is something of which to be ashamed.

Worry even if you really have some deep problems—need you also lose your looks? But do ask yourself whether you *really* have much to worry about.

Posture

It is common sense that a slack posture:

1 Makes you feel slack, mentally and physically.

2 Means that vital organs are not in the most healthy position in relation to each other.

3 Means that the lungs in particular are probably not able to expand fully when you breathe in.

4 Risks torso muscles getting out of condition.

5 Risks the accumulation of fat around the waist, tummy, and diaphragm.

6 Last, but not least, it absolutely ruins your appearance. The line of a garment must of necessity follow the line of the body wearing it.

Here are some tips for acquiring good posture

1 Without strain and in a way which feels natural to you, expand until you *feel* tall and straight and beautiful as you move about. (Notice that I say *feel* straight. The body cannot, of course, *be* straight—it is made of so many wonderful curves.)

2 When walking, gently but firmly and without strain, pretend that you are a sandwich that must be flattened a little, the front of your body being one side of the sandwich filling which must be flattened or squeezed. As you use your muscles to achieve this end, you will be amazed at the way in which your contours grow firmer and your posture improves.

3 Imagine your chest is attached to a pulley in the ceiling while your feet are firmly fixed to the floor, and the pulley is gently but firmly stretching you up.

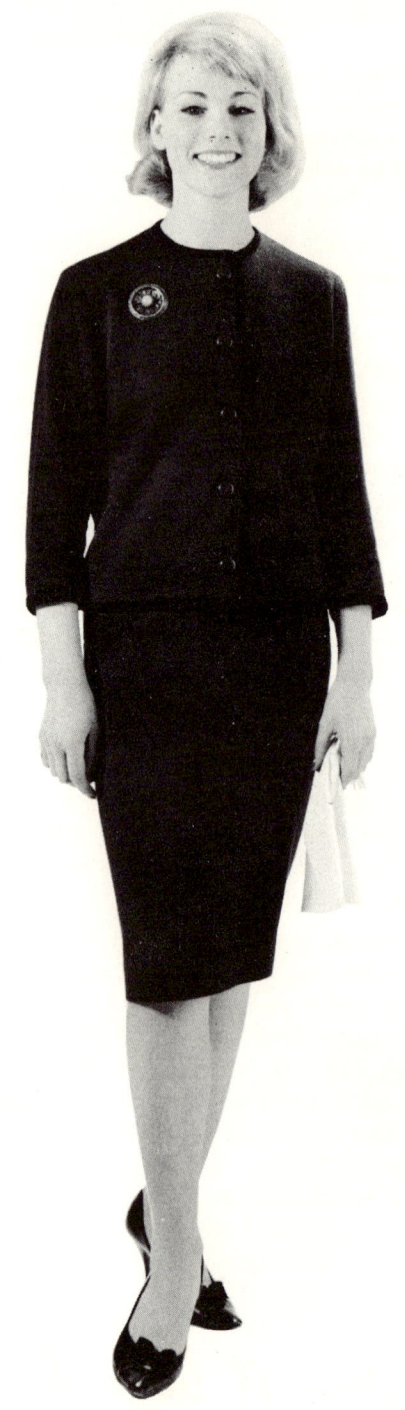

facial expression and posture 17

4 Look at yourself frontways in a full-length looking glass and check whether (*a*) your hips are level and (*b*) your shoulders are level. Your posture is not right if either are out of alignment. In addition, your shoulders should be well pulled down. Watch your neckline respond to the firm pulling down of shoulders.

5 Look at yourself sideways in a full-length looking glass and check for general straightness of line. The most important thing is to have the back of the head in alignment with the back, and if you observe that you are round-shouldered, then you can be sure that the head is being pushed forward. If your tummy protrudes too much, then expanding upwards out of the waist will help to flatten it, but when you do this, watch that the shoulders remain pulled down. Always see what an easy straightening of the back will do first.

6 In the privacy of your bedroom, watch all your movements as much as you can in the full-length looking glass. Dressing and undressing give you daily opportunities for this. Correct ungraceful hurried movements and notice that the more poised and graceful your movements, the more the body posture looks right. These things go together. Notice, too, that you never look right if your stance is either too slack or too tensed up. Particularly watch how graceful you look when stooping if you bend at the hip and knee joints rather than bending the back.

7 Take the daily opportunities offered, such as when waiting at a bus stop, on a platform, or standing when traveling, to check posture. Work from the feet upwards or from the head downwards (it doesn't matter much which way you do it), slowly and deliberately easing the body into a good position and allowing it to expand, as it were, to its full height.

I do hope you will get started right away on some of these ideas because in the next chapter I shall be explaining how to train yourself to walk from the hips, and before you can do that—

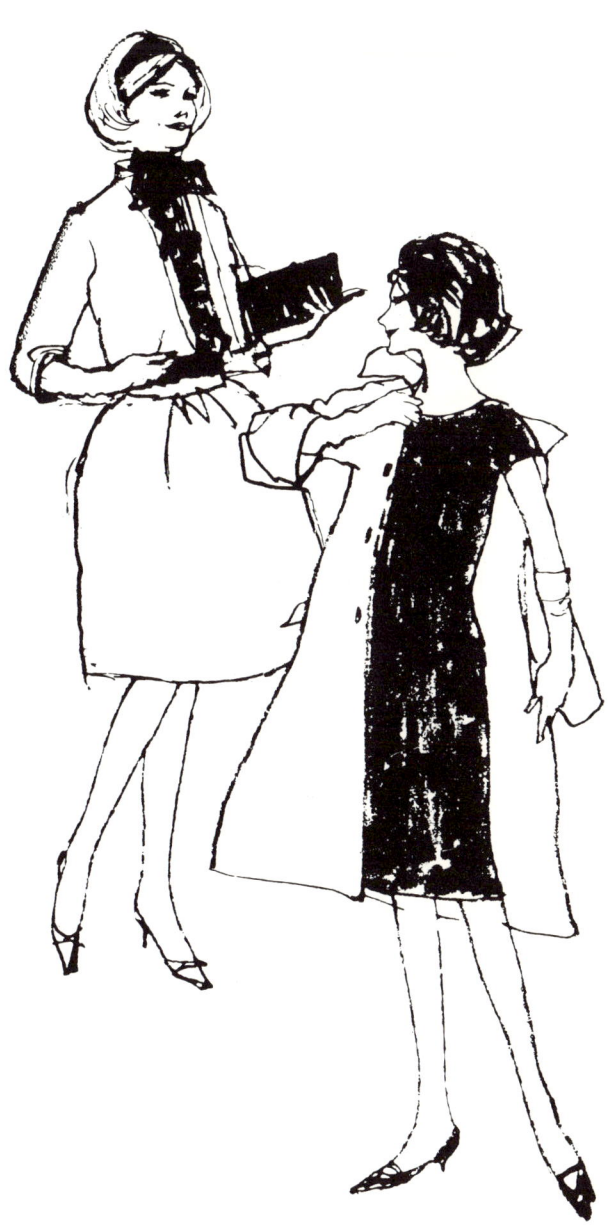

you must be able to walk in good posture

Things not necessarily noticed

Finally, here are one or two things to which the eye of the beholder does *not* necessarily jump.

irregular teeth

People may not notice these, but they may be puzzled by a peculiar smile, or no smile at all, if this is what you do in an effort at concealment.

scars

It is being petty-minded about yourself to think that people take one look at you and think: Ah! Scar on eyebrow (or wherever it is). They may in fact know you for years without noticing it. Meanwhile you may have been suffering quite unnecessary tortures of self-consciousness about it. I knew one girl who always seemed to be standing in a peculiar way when people were talking to her, and eventually I found out that she was just worried that a scar on her leg would be noticed. (As if it mattered even if it *were* noticed!) A little ordinary foundation cream or special scar cream can always be used in any case.

moles and freckles

Just stop moaning about them. *If* people notice them at all, they are really not critical of them, but just take them for granted.

large hands

Let them be beautifully cared for and used as exquisitely as if they were small and dainty.

large feet

Avoid light and bright shoes. Find neat footwear which by cunning line create an illusion of smallness and slenderness.

big ears

Wear hair to cover all, or some part of, the ears.

RIGHT *Sophia Loren. Her large, generous mouth contributes to her individuality.*

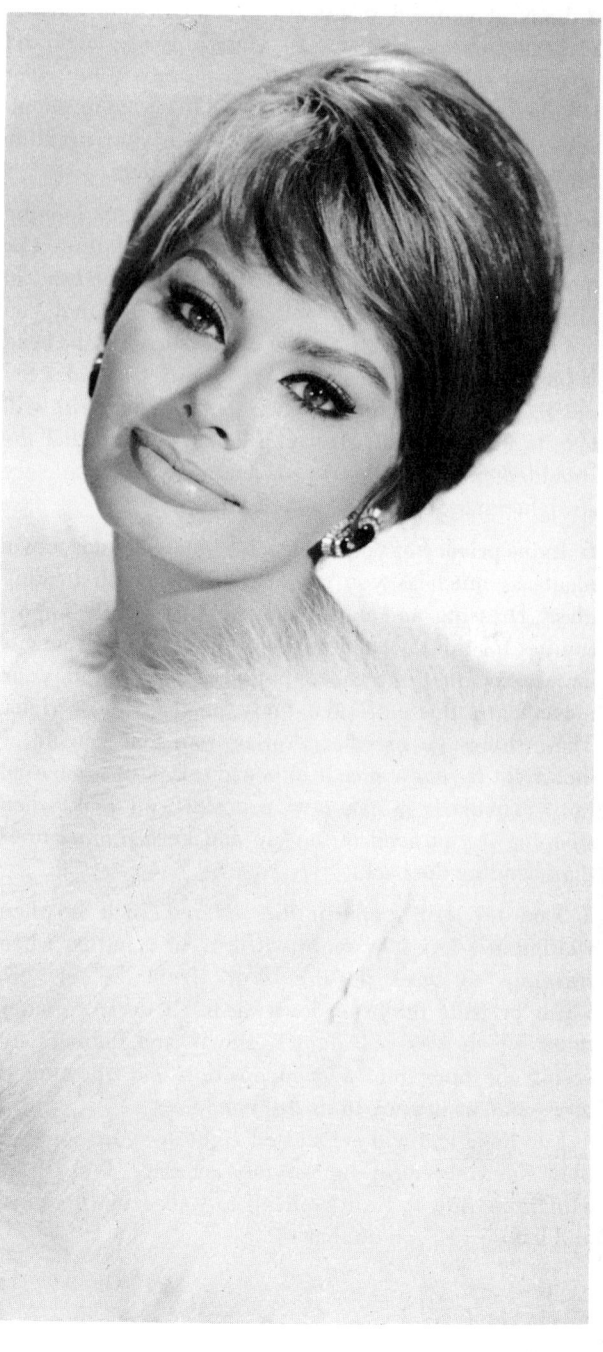

3 deportment

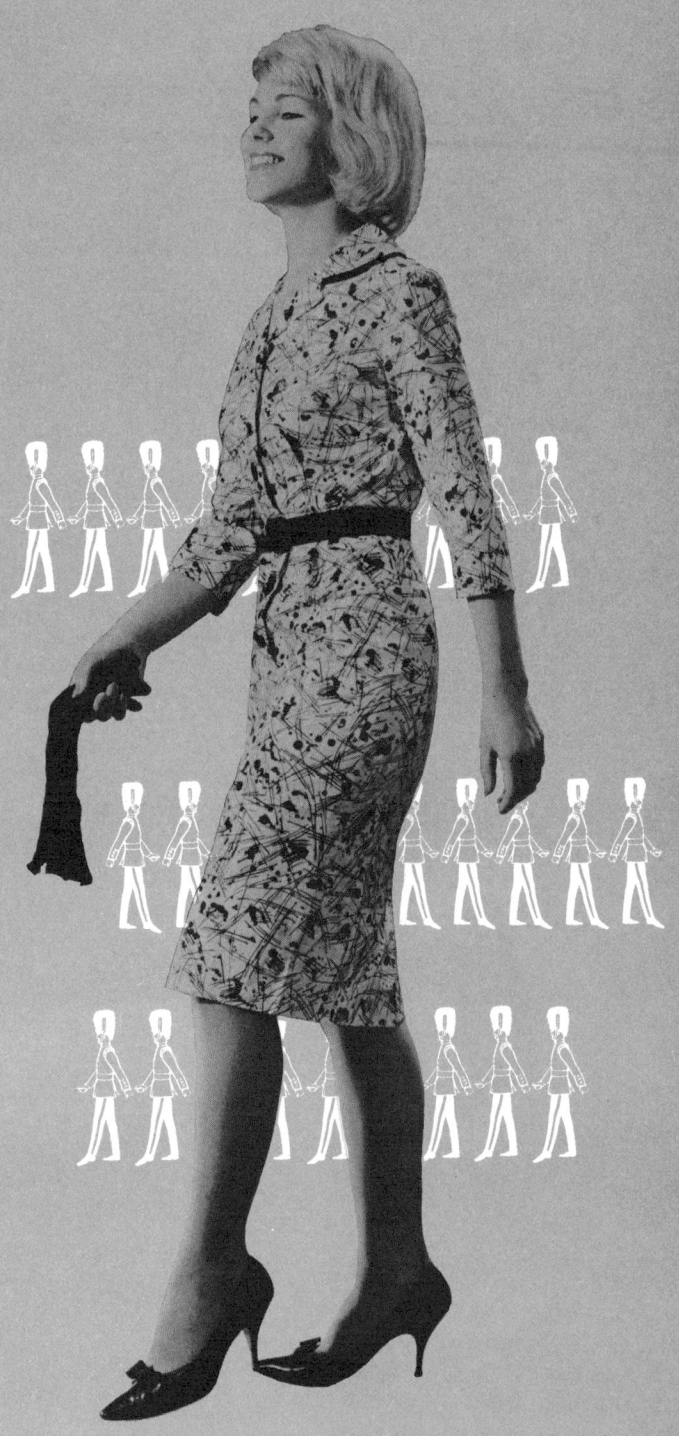

You are judged a great deal by the way you walk, sit, stand, and manage stairs, by your mannerisms, and by the way you move about generally.

Walking

Do you lurch forward with your whole body weight bearing down on each step?

Get the long-legged look by walking from the hip, legs leading, body weight following. The best way to train yourself to get the right relationship between body weight and step is to copy the ceremonial marching of soldiers on parade in which the forward foot pauses momentarily just in front of the other foot. You must have seen this in films or on television many times. The body weight should be held up a second on the pause, allowing the foot to complete its step unencumbered by the weight of the body. (This is where it is essential to be holding the body in good posture.) Once you have got the idea, cut out the pause and practice your new walking to the strains of a strict-tempo tango. The rhythm will inspire smoothness and grace. It is a rather lovely idea to walk in the street to the strains of some glorious music singing in your mind. (But only in quiet streets, please, not where there is traffic.)

Are you inherently ungainly, or jerky?

Although the ideas above will help, the only real cure for lack of gracefulness in movement is to join a class for rhythmic movement or for Modern Dancing. In this, you also learn about color, composition, expression, as well as acquiring a deeper knowledge of the music of the great composers.

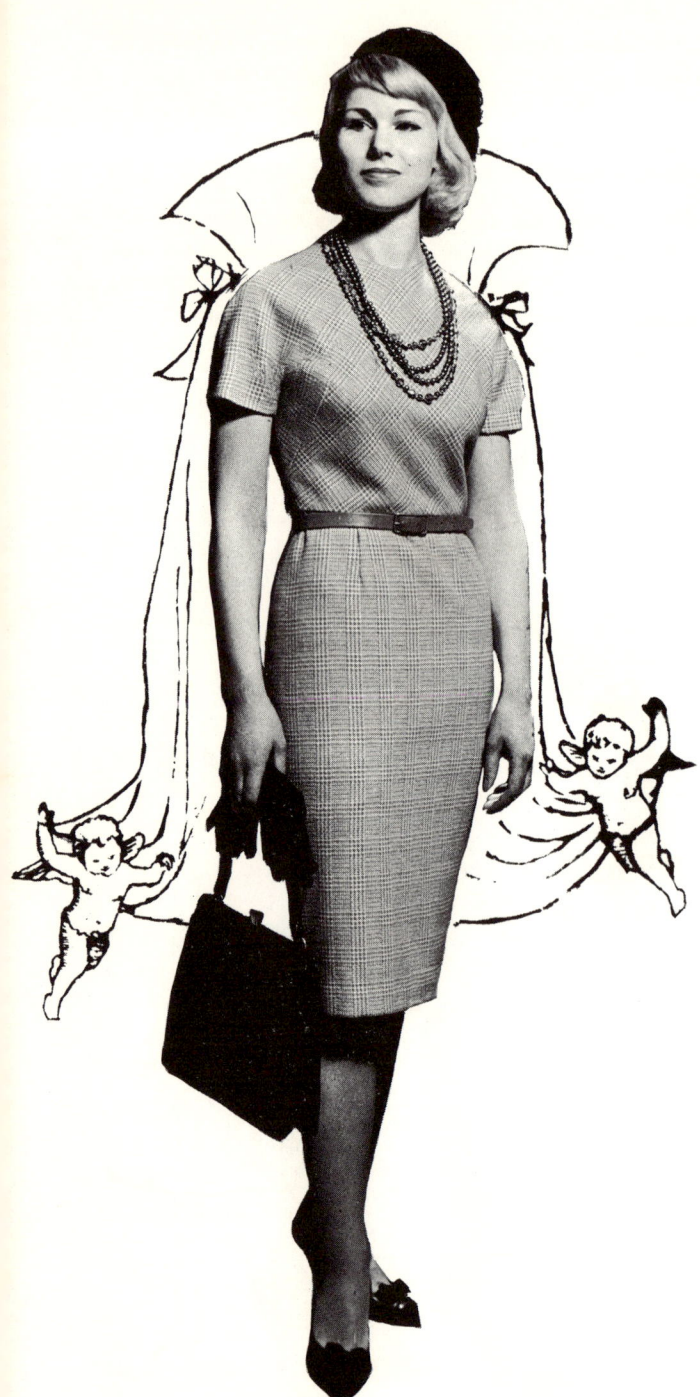

Do your shoulders move with each step?

Keep your shoulders firm and well pulled down. The whole torso should only be concerned with maintaining good posture, and no part of it should be trying to help with the business of stepping forward. In any case an undisciplined torso will spoil the line of your dresses.

Does your head crane forward?

Keep the back of the head in alignment with the back—this has already been mentioned among the points for acquiring good posture. But when you cross a room or a ballroom floor, move the head regally and graciously and at slow-motion pace from side to side, looking at the people there with interest. If you find this difficult, try imagining that you are a queen looking at her subjects. Nobody will know what you are thinking, but it will give you the right confident look. In any case, never enter a room or cross a floor thinking, "Oh dear, everybody is looking at *me*". Replace this thought by, "I am looking at *them*".

Are you gloriously unconscious of flailing arms, or of fussy hands?

Do you have one arm batting the air just because you happen to be carrying something a little heavy with the other?

Do you have a hearty, businesslike swing of the arm across the body, either from the shoulder or from the elbow?

For perfect poise, you should always be in complete control of arms and hands, and both should be used as beautifully and delicately as possible.

Do your toes turn out? Do they turn in? Does the toe part of your shoe wave in the air a little before it takes the ground?

Feet should go down straight, neither turned out nor turned in. Heel and toe should appear to go down together, although in fact the heel must go down a split

deportment 21

second first, but only a split second. If the ball of the foot is occasionally allowed to go down first, you will feel braked, and in addition it will look odd.

Do you overdo tightrope walking? *(do you move each foot on to the* OTHER SIDE *of the tight-rope?)*

Tightrope walk if you must, or if it just comes naturally to you, but the best placing of the feet is straight ahead —just on either side, as it were, of that straight rope.

And what about barefoot walking—at the swimming pool, on the beach! Do your toes curl up saying "we're not used to this"?

This is when the ball of the foot *should* reach the ground first—again only a split second before the rest of the foot. Just try it, and see if you don't acquire the grace of the traditional water carriers of old.

Standing

Too tired to hold yourself up?

Good posture is essential, but don't stand at attention. Introduce the slightest spiral into the body by placing one foot a little behind the other. It is best to take the weight on to the back foot, and then the front is ready for the takeoff. Study the position in front of your full-length looking glass. If you try placing the back foot at an angle of forty-five degrees to your other foot, you will see that you have achieved a position similar to that of a model at her moment of pause.

Do your arms hang tent-like from your shoulders with your hands looking lost and saying "we never know what to do with ourselves"?

Adopt *one or two* simple gestures—hands clasped lightly in front of you, one hand lightly in a pocket, graceful holding of handbag, one hand delicately touching a fold of a full-skirted dress, etc. Try it all out in front of your looking glass with each of your outfits. After practice, you will find that, like the model, you will use these movements naturally and unconsciously. As long as you don't overdo them, you will soon find that you are gaining exactly the right look of assurance.

Are you guilty of washerwoman arms? *(arms folded across the front of the body)*

If you are trying to hide your figure, then you are rather drawing attention to it. The position is bad for breathing, and it makes you look round-shouldered, apologetic and thoroughly ungraceful.

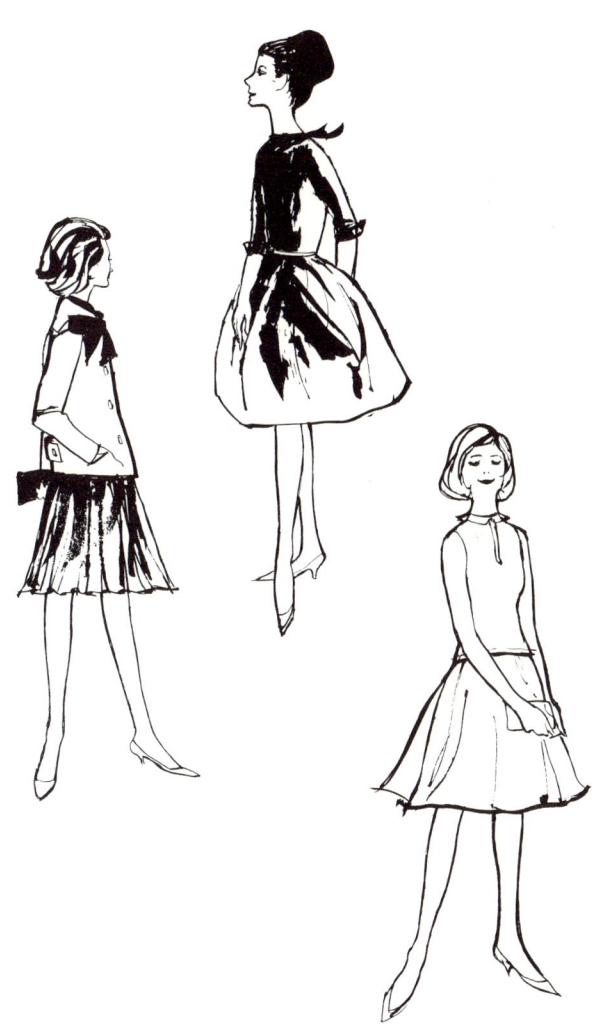

Sitting

Do your knees and ankles sag apart?

Do your feet droop away from each other at unattractive angles?

And, once again, are you just too tired to hold yourself up?

Keep your feet, ankles and knees together and, as much as possible, at the same angle.
Lolling around in a chair appearing tired looks frightful, and is extremely discourteous to those around you. If you need a rest, then pull yourself together until you can retire for a little while. Then spend fifteen minutes lying down, and indulge in some conscious and deep breathing, thinking of nothing but the breath and its health-giving properties.

If you sit with crossed legs, is there an ungainly twelve inches between ankles, and is one calf being bulged out?

Sitting with crossed legs is, strictly speaking, bad form. But we all do it. To train yourself to do it attractively, place a chair in front of the full-length looking glass. Watch yourself as you take a seat and then try crossing the legs just above the knee. Bring the ankles and feet together, both feet pointing in the same direction. This can look absolutely bewitching, whether the legs are on the straight or on a slant.

As you are about to sit down, do you pass your hands right over your seat in an effort to smooth down your skirt?

This is not a gesture for grown-ups. Instead, pause a moment to allow the skirt to fall between you and the chair. Bending the knees a little forward helps. Even if you are engaged in conversation as you sit, you should be aware of what is happening to your skirt. Tight skirts should not be allowed to slide too high above the knees, so that they have repeatedly to be pulled down. Full skirts will need placing to each side so that they don't frumpishly drown the legs and feet.

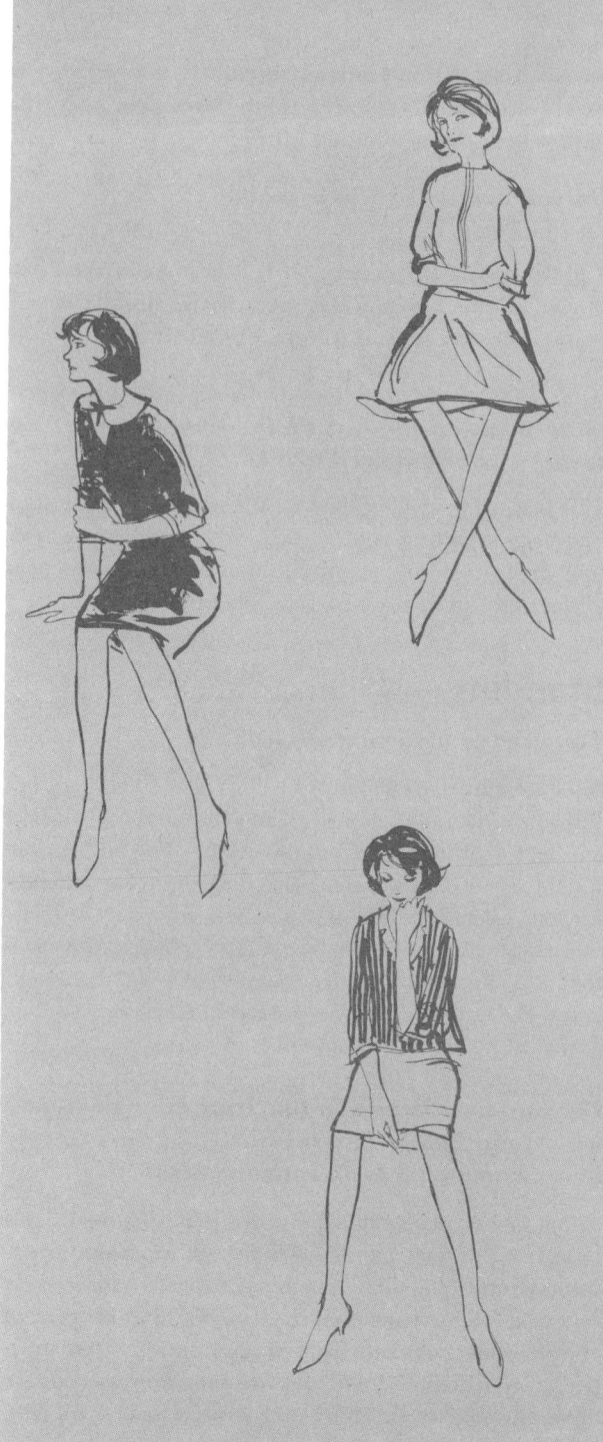

Do you hitch up your skirt in the manner of a man pulling at the crease of his trousers?

If you can, manage without hitching up a straight skirt. Ideally, of course, the lining should take any strain, and not the skirt. If you feel you must hitch it up, then do it by placing the palms of the hands at the hip level and ease the skirt up from there. This looks feminine and French.

Do you get into and out of deep seats, deck chairs and cars like a struggling baby elephant?

Take your time and do it all in easy stages. When getting down, drop your weight first on to the edge of the seat, then ease back in one or two stages. Reverse this when getting up, easing yourself to the edge of the seat before attempting to rise. Thus you rise beautifully and vertically and avoid the pitfall of trying to move both forward and upward in one sprawly movement.

And what about the front seat of cars? Do you straddle in with one foot first—looking pretty ungainly and stretching your skirt?

Wise girls get in backwards. Let your hands help a little as you get on to the edge of the seat, then, *keeping feet and knees together*, rock back a little while you draw in the feet, and then rock forward as you tuck them into the front of the car. Do it all slowly and unhurriedly and you will look enchanting and poised at a moment when the majority of women look their worst.

Last, but certainly not least, how do you sit for working? Do you allow the weight of your body to rest on the fleshy part of the seat and thighs?

Sitting for hours each day like this will certainly tend to make you look flabby and not put you in the best position for normal full deep breathing. Come to the edge of a hard chair or stool, find the bones in your seat, and sit on them. Feel the hardness of bone meeting the hardness of hard chair. You'll discover this is the easy way to keep your back straight and to give you flexibility of movement while working.

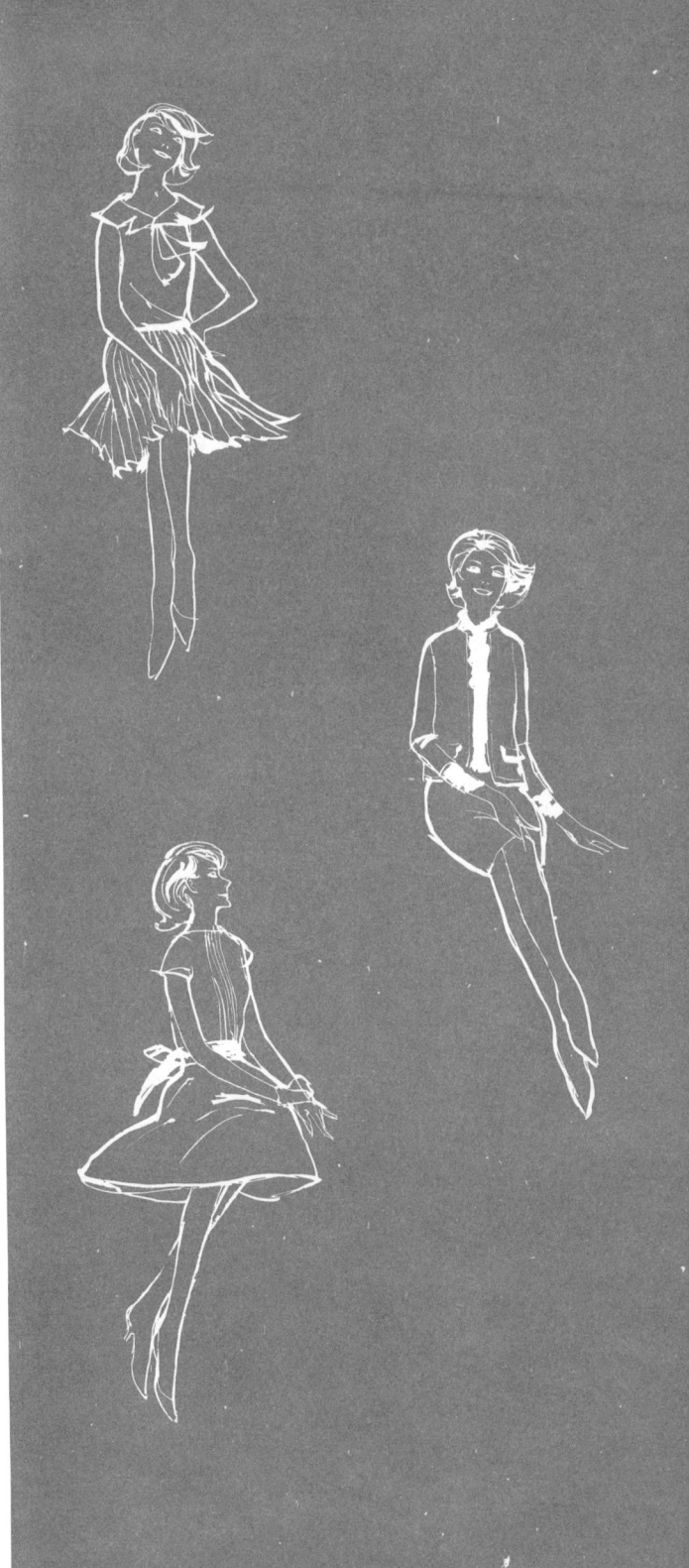

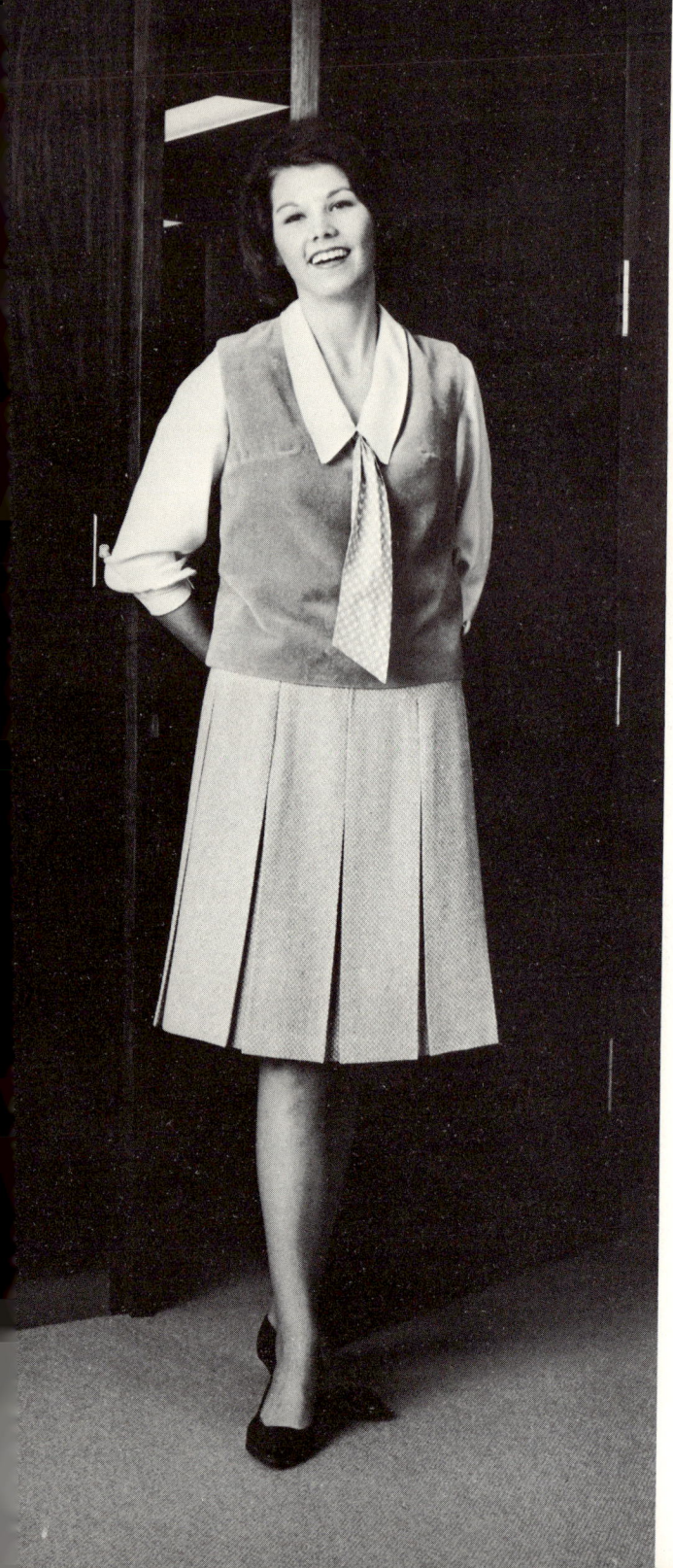

Entrances

Do you creep round the door looking at the woodwork or the handle, then at the floor or the ceiling?

Or perhaps you rush in making a commotion, letting the door swing wildly out of control?

And then maybe you start talking nineteen to the dozen regardless of whether the person to whom you are speaking is (a) speaking to someone else, (b) speaking on the telephone, or (c) adding up a column of figures?

The secret of a good entrance is to come in without commotion, closing the door with both arms behind you so that you are looking into the room. The picture is even more attractive if you slide yourself into the middle of the door so that you are framed, as it were. Look at the person or persons in the room with a smile.

Exits

Do you creep up to a door and creep round it like a shy child?

Or perhaps you swing the door wildly, not caring whether or not it closes with a bang?

When reaching for the door handle, do you sag back, losing posture and thrusting your seat out backwards?

The secret of a good exit is to walk to the door unhurriedly, keeping tall and straight as you open the door, and at the moment of disappearing, turning the head with a smile, or even just turning the head slightly. Don't overdo this. Close the door efficiently and quietly.

Photograph by King Beach

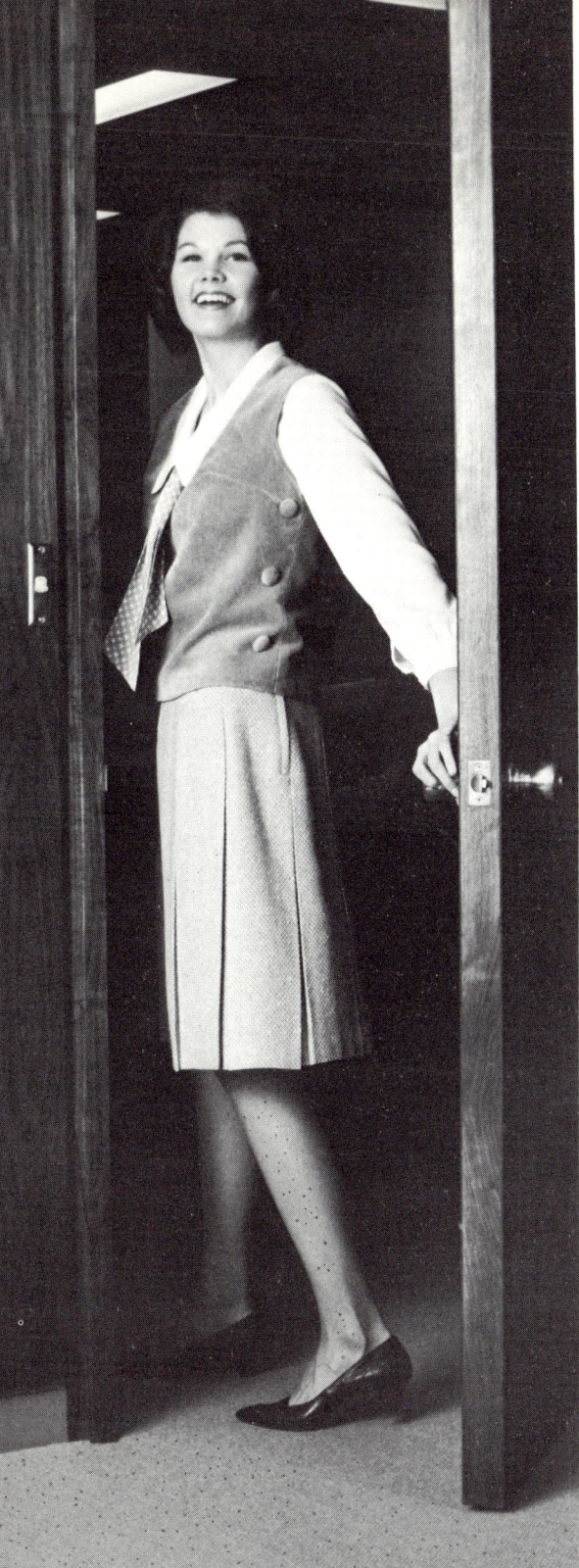

Stairs

Do you go pigeon-toed?

Do you plonk down the whole of the foot?

Do you allow your seat to assume a near sitting position?

Does your seat take on strange rolls and curves?

Do your feet and legs do all the work?

Does the whole thing lack grace and become a weary effort?

Do you gather up your full-length evening gown like an ecstatic child in a party dress?

Do you come down hanging on to the handrail?

Do you put the heel down first?

Do you lift your long skirt when descending?

Young woman, you should go up those stairs like a bird, treading on the ball of the foot only. With exquisite fingers you should raise that heavenly gown only an inch or two from your impeccable slippers. And try using the right muscles for the job, that is to say, the muscles in the seat. After all, the whole body is a weighty thing and when it comes to giving it a vertical lift, the strong seat muscles which extend well down into the thigh are right for the job. Thus no unnecessary strain will be put upon the more delicate muscles of the knees, ankles, and feet. Furthermore, I suppose I ought to add that many an expert advises using the whole of the foot when ascending stairs, but frankly, this can look stodgy.

You should come down like a dream too, but slowly, taking your time, and feeling for each stair with the ball of the foot. Using the ball of the foot (and not the heel at all) when descending is even more important than for ascending, because if the heel of your shoe makes contact with the stair first, then, as your body follows on, its full weight may be thrown on to the toe part of your foot, which by now may be in midair over

Photograph by King Beach

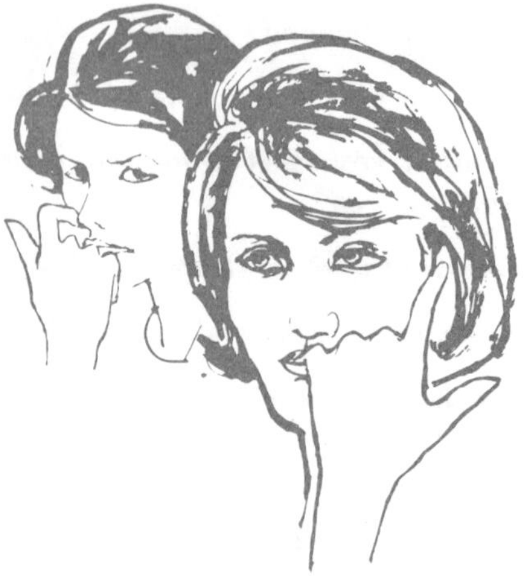

the edge of the stair. Very dangerous! Finally, if you want to do the job one hundred per cent correctly, then don't use the handrail and don't lift your gown at all—it is supposed to be taking a forward impetus created by your descent, and your feet are then safely inside—as in a tent.

However, let's come down to earth. Safety first is the right motto for negotiating stairs, especially the difficult or narrow ones.

Mannerisms

Do you tweak (fingers and fingernails), twiddle (rings and back hair), scratch (anywhere), fiddle (with anything), pull faces, chew gum, ruminatively rub your face?

Do you gesticulate when talking?

Be your own severest critic for a while—and find out what your mannerisms are. That irresistible tickle on the end of the nose can be dealt with by a delicate rub from a spotless feminine handkerchief or tissue (which ought anyway to be easily available in case you sneeze). That itchy scalp is Nature's way of telling you it's out of condition. General fidgetiness can perhaps be traced to the fact that you never allow yourself proper time to get ready, or to get anywhere, or to relax. Finally, gesticulating attracts undue attention.

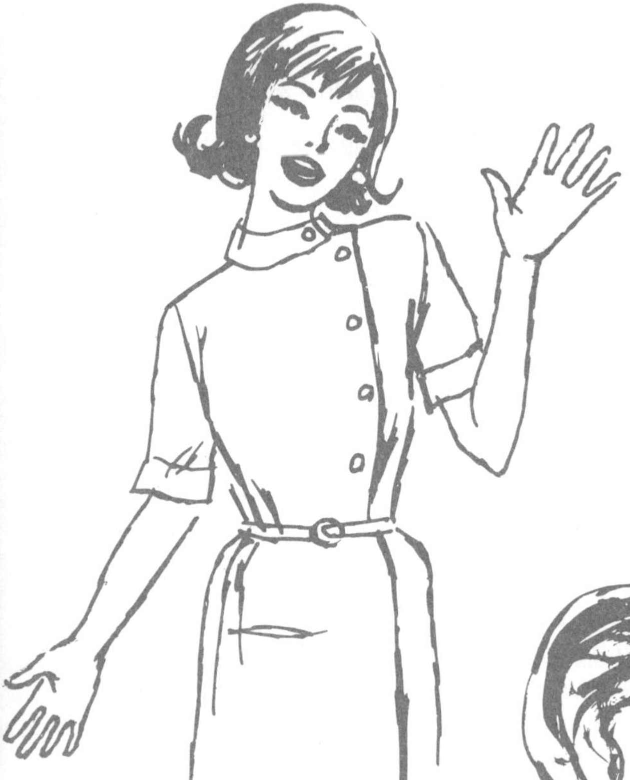

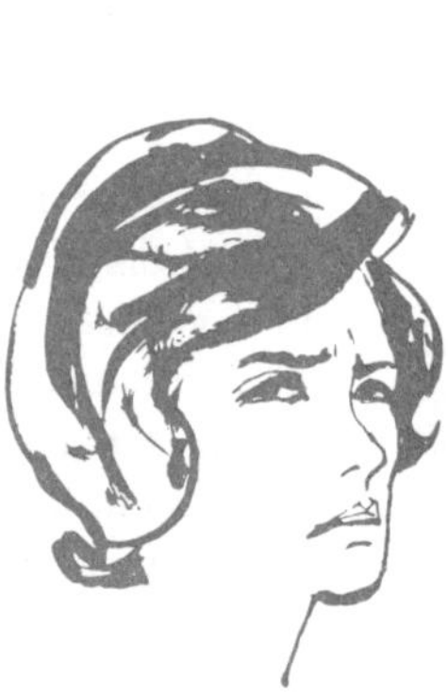

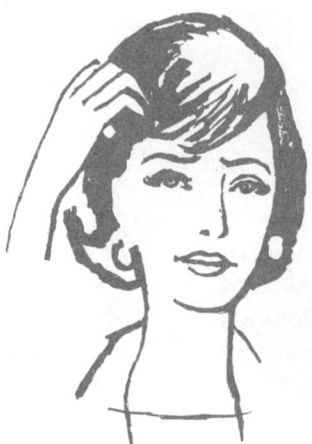

4 figure, my threefold attack

Quietly, calmly and *without fuss and quite gradually* organize your life so that the threefold attack is part and parcel of everyday living, and decide *now* that you are not going to lose your figure as you grow older.

What is my threefold attack?

1 *Using the body in all its normal everyday activities beautifully and correctly. The chapter on deportment has already given you a general picture of this.*
2 *Eating to live (not living to eat).*
3 *Exercising, but particularly becoming an enthusiastic walker, and breathing deeply and rhythmically.*

Eating to live

If you fill your stomach with such things as cookies, chocolates, sweets, cakes, buns, pastries, white bread, and cups of tea or coffee, it may well be that you do not feel any pangs of hunger and yet you could be undernourished. Today, scientists tell us about the miracle that is the human body, the way it works, the chemicals it needs to work efficiently, what foods these chemicals are found in, and in what proportion we need these foods. Day in, day out, there are articles in the women's magazines, articles in newspapers, and booklets galore, translating this knowledge into everyday eating habits. *I have come to the conclusion that this magnificent knowledge is read, often by those who most need it, like so much fiction —and the advice never followed.* Perhaps this applies to you? A famous dietitian once said "Eat what your body *needs* first, then eat what you like." This, you will discover, is a very wise but tongue-in-cheek remark, because when you have eaten what you need of

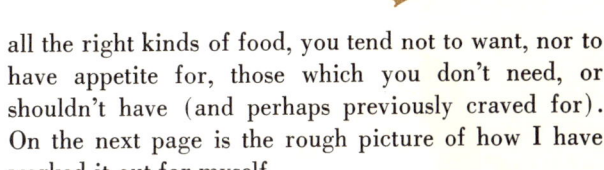

all the right kinds of food, you tend not to want, nor to have appetite for, those which you don't need, or shouldn't have (and perhaps previously craved for). On the next page is the rough picture of how I have worked it out for myself.

I consider:

1 That canned, processed, and frozen foods are for emergency use only.
2 That fruits, vegetables, and salads should be eaten *fresh*.
3 That when eating away from home, it is better to avoid discussing diet, and that it is best to say one would like this or that (keeping as near as possible to one's considered diet) giving no explanations.
4 That thorough mastication and eating in a calm frame of mind are vitally important.
5 That suitable snacks when hungry are:
(*a*) Cream cheese and raisins
(*b*) An apple
(*c*) An orange
(*d*) Radishes, walnuts, and cheese
(*e*) A prune or two (just washed, not soaked). This is an ideal snack for the slimmer.

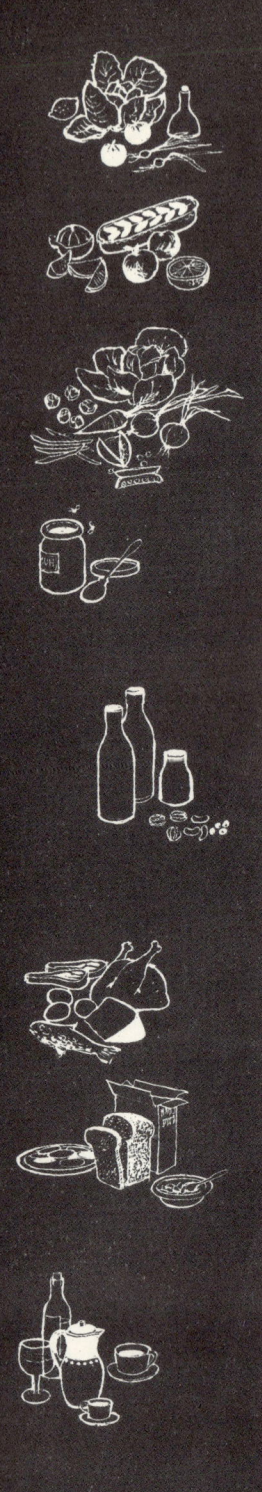

Two-thirds intake each day drawn from the following:

Salads in season   *With fresh lemon juice, olive oil, parsley, onion*

Fruits in season   *Basically two apples and two oranges a day and perhaps some dried fruits (raisins, prunes, apricots)*

Vegetables in season   *Especially the green ones*
Sparingly of root vegetables

Honey   *In strict moderation, say one or two teaspoonful a day (and entirely taking the place of jams, marmalades)*

Milk, Yogurt, Nuts

One-third intake each day drawn from the following:

Cheese
Eggs
Fish
Flesh
Fowl

I get my main protein from milk, nuts, eggs, and cheese. I suppose you will also get yours from fish, flesh, and fowl, but I've never so much as tasted these myself.

Bread
Biscuits
Cereals
Wheat germ

Keeping to such products as wholewheat bread and biscuits, pumpernickel bread, and whole grain cereals.

Tea and Coffee   *Ideally, one would be better without these altogether. However, this is a tall order. I compromise and have them in strict moderation.*

(f) Celery and cheese

(g) Tomato juice (the one canned food I allow myself)

6 That if you have spots, a muddy complexion, or if you're overweight, then eating on the lines I have set out should help enormously. (If it has been suggested to you that these troubles are caused because of your adolescence, then realize that this period of swift mental and physical growth can bring disturbances in the system—which will pass. Sometimes this problem gives rise to friction with parents, and, should this apply to you, couldn't you and your parents agree to laugh it off for the passing phase that it is?)

7 That if you need to put on weight, then in addition to eating on the lines set out, you can eat plentifully of the types of food on which the slimmer must go carefully—milk, ice cream, honey, dried fruits, bananas, nuts, rich cheeses, etc. But avoid the pitfall of thinking you can eat anything. Fried foods, chocolates, pastries, and buns may increase your weight, but it may not be the right kind of weight. Keep roughly to a preponderance of salads, fruits, and vegetables to maintain the balance of chemicals, and then you are doing what you can to build up firm flesh and a clear skin.

Exercising

First of all jot down your main measurements—bust, waist, widest part (usually at the curve of the seat, sometimes at thigh or tummy level), and height (in stocking feet). Now don't be misled. You may have the same measurements as B.B. (Brigitte Bardot), and yet your figure might not look the least bit like hers. Knowing your measurements is not enough. For an understanding of your figure, turn an analytical eye upon it in the looking glass. Check the following:

(a) *Does your tummy take on an outward bulge?*

(b) *Is your seat too prominent?*

(c) *Is there a spare tire at your diaphragm?*

(d) *Is your torso short?*

(e) *Is your torso long?*

(f) *Is your torso wide—and* **where is it wide,** *at the shoulders, the back, or the hips?*

The first three (which are figure faults) can probably be cured. The last three (which are more to do with the basic architecture of your body) must be kept firmly in mind when building up your own dress sense.

Exercising is not a thing apart in your life, but part and parcel of everyday living. Working through your day, I should like to think that you come to a joyful appreciation of all the opportunities offered. First there is the exercise inherent in the morning toilet (dealt with in the chapter on Grooming). Then there is the whole field of deportment already dealt with. And then there are the many opportunities for *walking*, five minutes here, ten minutes there, possibly adding up to about two hours a day in all. It is by becoming an enthusiastic walker, together with breathing rhythmically and deeply, that you can learn to *throw off fatigue, have more energy, and be mentally calm.*

the way to do it

1 Only when alone. If you are with others, give them your full attention.

2 Not on busy roads because you should then be keeping your mind on the traffic.

3 Wear walking shoes. If these are not right with your outfit, then change temporarily into flat heels, which you could carry with you. Or sometimes you can compromise with shoes that have a smart, neat, not too high heel and that are right with the outfit.

4 Walk with a good posture, and from the hip.

5 Count the number of paces you take to breathe in. Take the *same number* of paces to breathe out. If you find that you are only counting up to four or six, here is a clear indication that you are not breathing deeply enough. One really simple way of getting yourself to breathe properly is to imagine you are taking air from a deep well, and then having to push it back again.

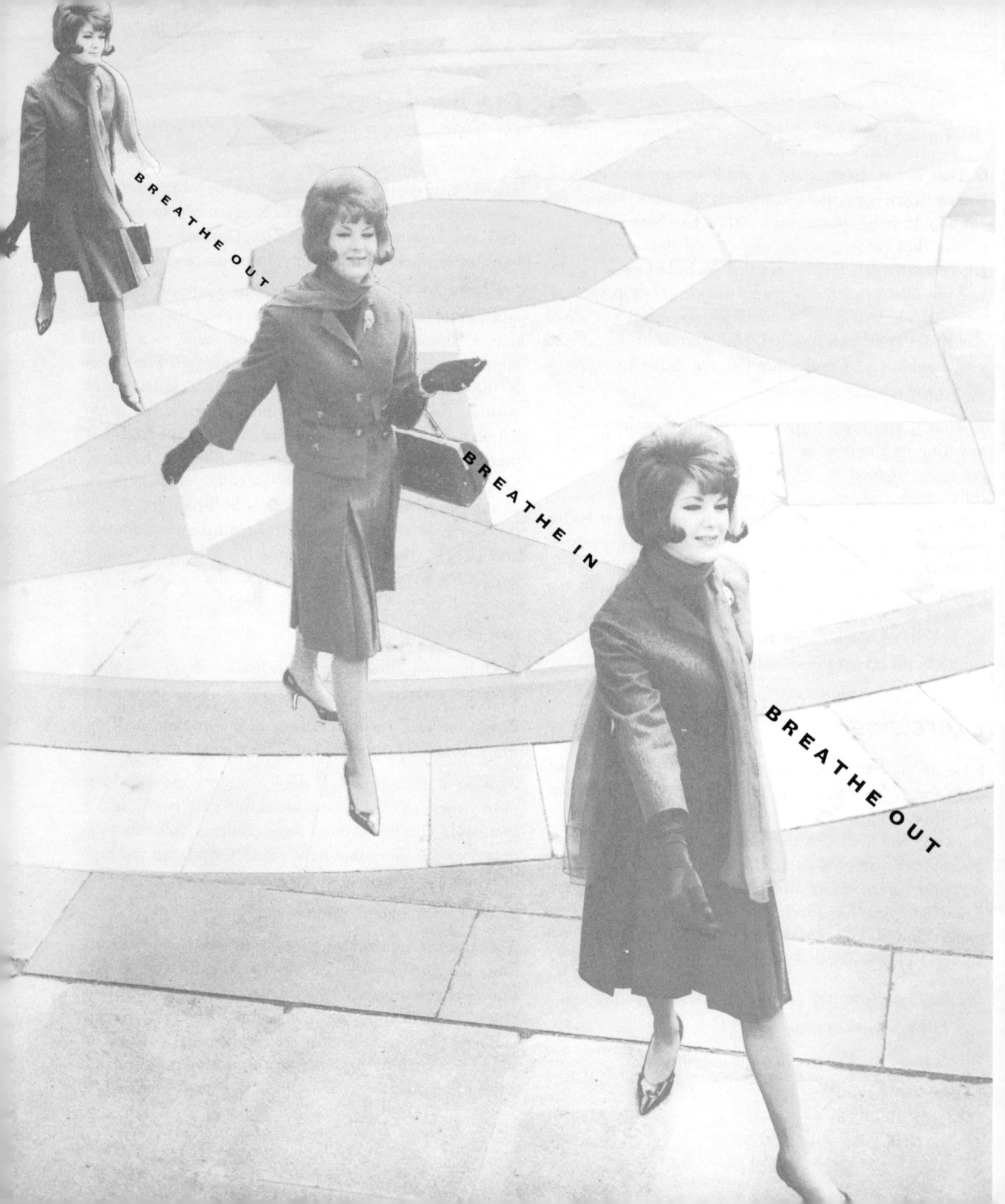

6 Think of nothing but the walking and breathing (except perhaps reveling in the sun, wind, or rain). Work, problems, worries, should all be dismissed for the time being with the thought that you will return to them with a fresh mind when the walking is over.

the reasons for doing it

1 Because fresh air, deep breathing, and exercise are as vital to your health and energy as calm relaxed sleep.

2 Because you need the refresher during the normal timetable of your busy day.

3 Because once you are walking in the fresh air, the deep rhythmic breathing ensures that you are getting the maximum benefit from it.

4 Because in breathing deeply, your lungs are being used fully, not merely half used, and more oxygen is being brought into the body.

5 Because the deep, slow breathing out means that the process of elimination on the outgoing breath is more thorough.

6 Because the giving up, as it were, of the whole being to movement, breathing, and atmosphere, is both mentally and physically refreshing.

Once you have accepted exercise into the normal pattern of your day, then all that remains is to devote a daily five or ten minutes to the resculpturing of your body where necessary. As in the case of diets, there is wonderful information given in women's magazines, beauty books, and the woman's page of daily newspapers, and if you set about it you can make quite a collection of the type of figure correction exercise you know you particularly need. A model with the right professional approach to her work would undoubtedly also give herself a top-to-toe exercise routine each morning. She must not only maintain her figure, but must also be in good physical condition. You can well imagine the demand made on muscles in her job.

The head

Exercising the neck by bending the head forward and backward and rolling from side to side is helpful in maintaining easy head movements. These movements are a daily *must*, for the model who is expected to move her head with regal poise in a fashion show or to hold her head in profile at the sharpest possible angle to the shoulders for a photograph.

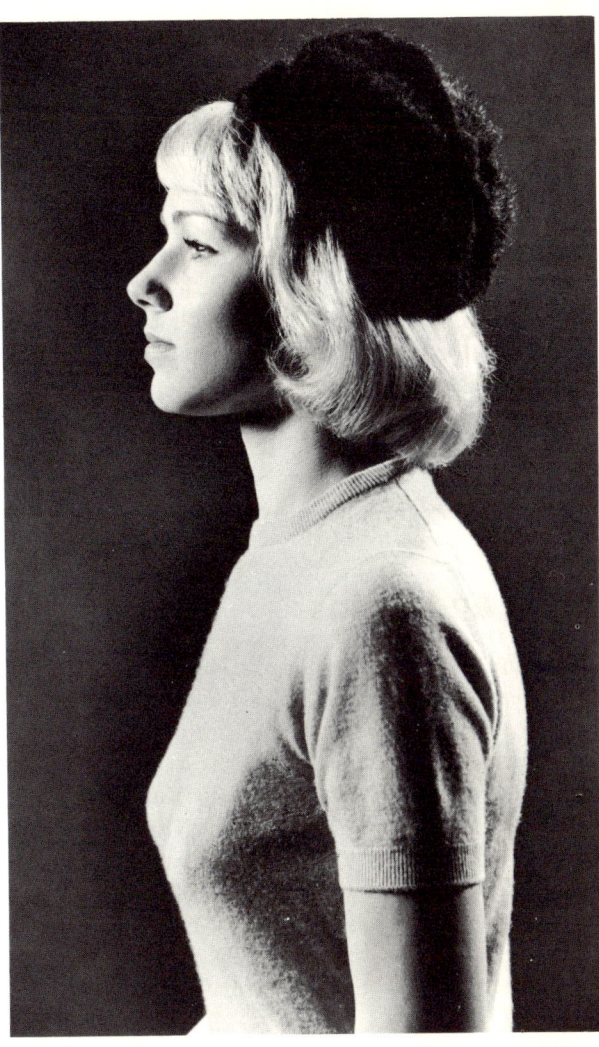

The eyes

Looking up and down, and from side to side (at eye level) can help to maintain mobility of eye muscles. These movements should be done quite slowly, gently, without any sense of strain, and with the head and shoulders kept quite still. Woe betide the model who is unable to change the direction of her eyes without at the same time changing the position of her head.

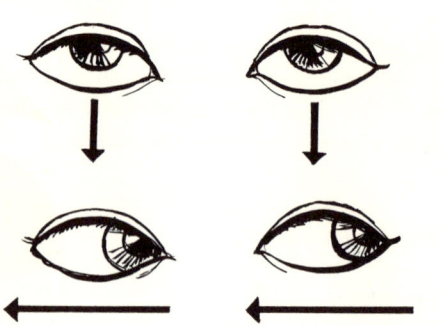

Arms and shoulders

Rhythmic arm circling helps to give grace and strength to the arms and shoulders. Try with arms singly, arms alternately, as well as arms working together. Rhythmic circling should start quite gently and slowly, and gradually work up speed and vigor as the shoulder becomes drawn into the movement—which should be felt right to the fingertips. Work out something for yourself to a strict-tempo waltz.

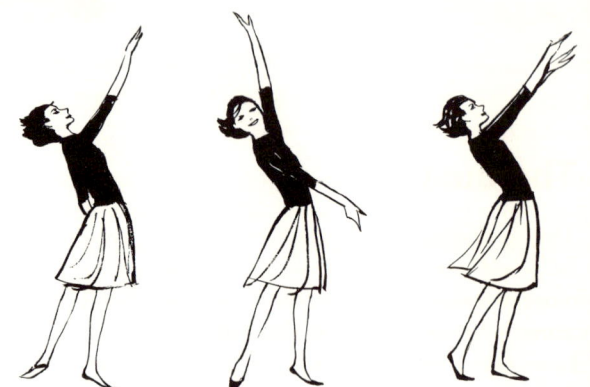

Arms and hands

Allow any lovely music to inspire some hand and arm movements. If this doesn't work for you, then imitate the movements of flames, trees, softly falling leaves, skimming water, or simply try stirring the air in figure-eight patterns in all directions with softly separated fingers. You will have seen for yourself that the model in the fashion picture always has her arms and hands beautifully placed. In a live fashion show she is expected to use arms and hands in the most exquisite manner from her moment of entrance, all the way up and down the platform to the last split second of her exit.

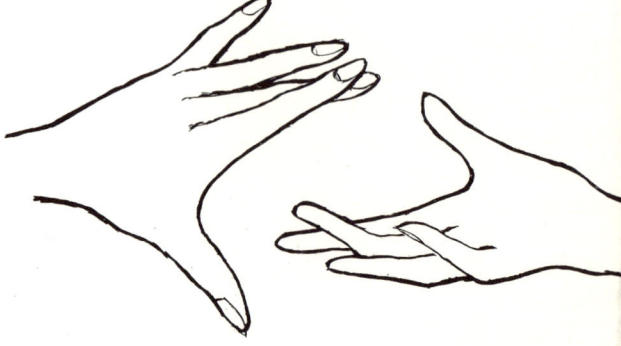

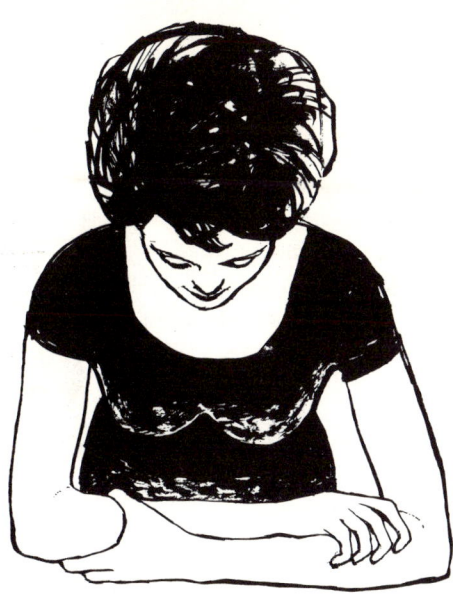

The bust

This is *the* bust exercise which is generally accepted to be beneficial for any type. Its aim is to tone the bust muscles, thereby encouraging better contour. Hold your arms in front of you at shoulder level. Bend both elbows and with each hand take a firm grip of the loose flesh midway between elbow and wrist of the other arm. Now, keeping your wrists rigid and straight *push* the flesh on each side up towards the elbow until it can't be pushed any further and a sense of braking is reached. When you feel a responsive movement in the bust muscle at the (quite vigorous) moment of braking, you will know you are doing the exercise correctly. Do this about 20 times.

Tense, straight, back-circling of the arms is one of the best exercises aimed at *bust development*. Clenched fists will help you to create the tension yourself (without the aid of something heavy in each hand), and the exercise will achieve more if you are breathing in on the away movement and breathing out on the return movement.

Tension should also be created in this exercise aimed at *reducing* the bust. Hold both hands out in front of the shoulders in the position for vertical clapping. Regard one hand as the most immovable object of all time, and the other as the greatest of all irresistible forces, so that when the latter moves up to the former (completing a clapping position), a strong tension is set up. Change the function of each hand after, say, five efforts—so that the exercise is completed an equal number of times on each side of the chest.

I am warning you, however, that busts tend to be very slow in responding to improvement exercises, and there is no guarantee that they will respond at all. But you have nothing to lose by trying. In any case the bust exercises are also good for the shoulders, shoulderblades, and arms.

If you tend to be slight-busted, wear a brassiere that will accentuate and give uplift, and console yourself with the thought that your figure will probably look younger longer (because it is never likely to reach matronly proportions). And let me remind you that prima ballerinas are invariably slight-busted, and that top models are tall and slight—and they are, after all, considered the acme of elegance.

If you tend to be overdeveloped, wear a brassiere that gives very firm control, and should you go on a slimming diet, then, at the same time, be sure to indulge in bust-toning and bust-reducing exercises.

The waist and diaphragm

Any side-bending will help to slenderize the waist area, but side-bending together with stretching is best. Stand with your feet a little apart and your arms straight up. Then stretch the torso upwards *before* bending sideways. The rhythm would go something like this—stretch-and-stretch-and-bend-and-bend-sideways-to-the-left, relax to the normal position; and then take the same rhythm, bending this time to the right. The exercise is equally beneficial from a good sitting position.

Another good diaphragm and waist exercise can be described as vigorous deep swinging. Stand with the feet a little apart, and, bending only from the waist, sweep the ground in front of you with just the tips of the fingers as both arms execute a parallel, pendulum-like swing. Allow the swing to become deeper and farther out at the sides as you go along.

There is no doubt that *everything* you wear, from a sack to a blouse and skirt to a bathing costume, looks better if you have a trim waist and flat diaphragm. Incidentally, when wearing belts, avoid notching them so tightly that the flesh is bulged out above and below.

Tummy

There are any number of exercises for keeping a flat tummy. Still one of the best is done lying flat on the back and, with legs and feet in the air, bicycling. Naturally, the feet and legs get exercise at the same time. I have developed the exercise in this way: The body position is flat on the back with the arms outstretched, palms upwards. The movement is raising both legs as high as possible from the hip and cycling eight times. Then with legs still up in the air, place them together and lower them slowly to the ground to a count of eight. While the legs are making the slow descent, stretch up slowly with the arms until they finish meeting on the floor above the head. At this point relax the entire body and start again.

If a model can't keep a flat tummy, she might just as well give up the profession. Should your tummy con-

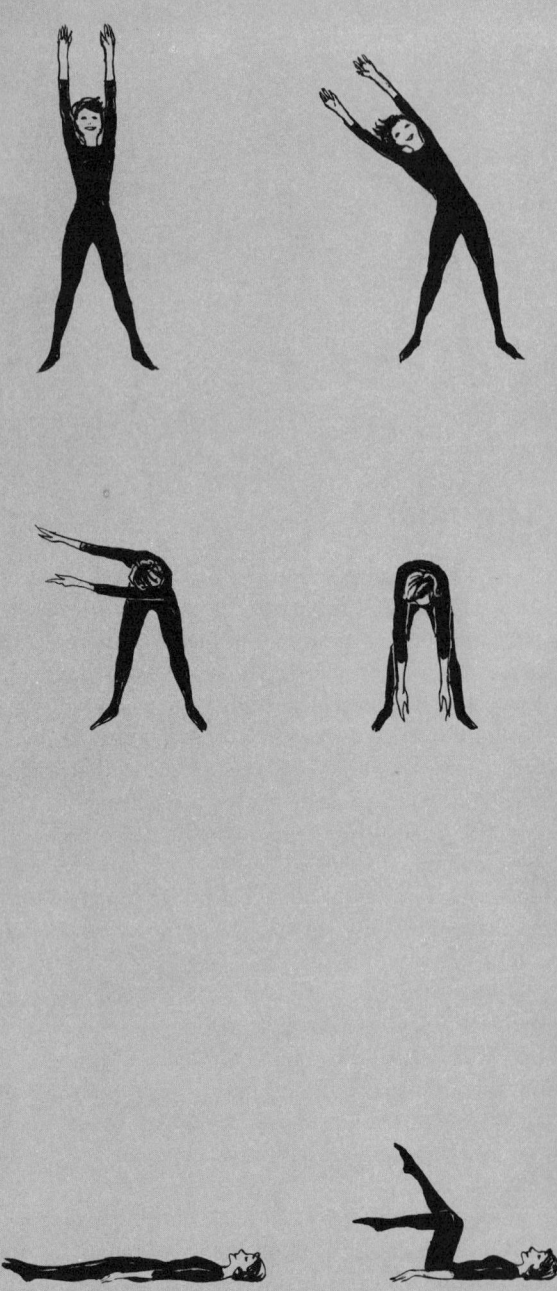

tinue to bulge or be too big despite good posture and exercises, then try (*a*) drinking less (if you are having more salads, green vegetables, and fruits in your diet, then you are introducing liquid into the system in a very natural way, and probably you don't *need* so much water, fruit juice, tea, coffee, etc.); (*b*) drinking only between meals (long drinks taken immediately after main meals do in some cases cause distension).

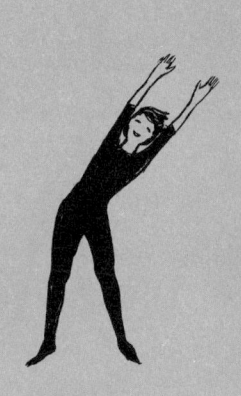

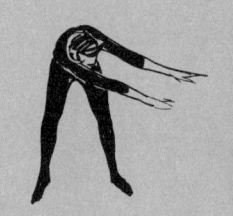

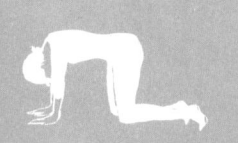

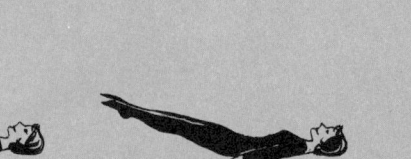

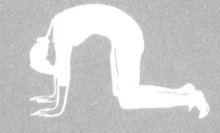

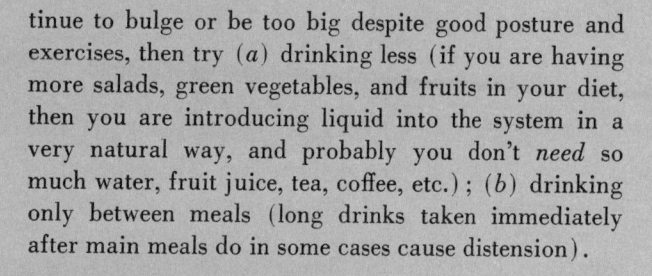

Here is another quite different tummy exercise. Kneel on all fours, with thighs and arms parallel with each other and supporting the torso. Keep the head relaxed downwards between the arms. Now arch the back slowly (rather like a cat), thus drawing in the tummy, then slowly release the tummy until the back is hollowed. (The drawing in of the tummy should of course also be done in the normal course of your day every time you bend forward.)

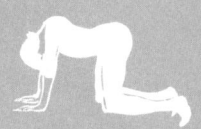

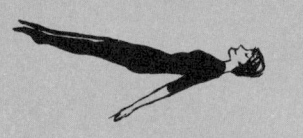

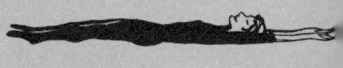

Seat and tummy

Try tightening up the seat slowly and deliberately, and then releasing it equally slowly and deliberately. If, as you do this, you let your hands move from the seat to the outer thigh and then to the tummy, you will realize that the tightening up of the large buttock muscles has a firming effect in these three parts of the body. You will remember that in the chapter on deportment, when talking about going up stairs, I recommended that you should use the muscles in the seat for lifting the body. In addition, use these muscles as often as convenient when walking and standing. Your ambition should be that your seat should forever be a small, round, firm object, and not a flabby, loose, spreading one, and these ideas—in addition to the eating of all the right foods—should help you to achieve that ambition.

Thighs and legs

Hold on to the back of a chair and give your legs (first one and then the other) pendulum movements, keeping the leg straight and in a straight swing (*not* the ballet type of leg movement). Clear the ground with the swinging leg. This simple movement exercises the thigh muscles at front and back and strengthens the lower part of the back. Be sure to keep the torso in a good, easy, firm posture, while the legs do all the work. If you are still struggling to walk from the hip this exercise may help you with that too.

Feet and legs

Skipping, running, little stiff jumps on the ball of the foot, are all wonderful for strengthening the feet and legs. And walking barefoot on springy turf or on the beach is fine for the well-being of the feet. One very good foot exercise is done sitting on the ground with hands resting on the ground a little way out from the body at each side and the feet about a foot apart—then, using both feet simultaneously, move them towards each other in a downward circle and then away from each other in a downward circle. This is rather like a downward circling figure-eight. Do this, say eight times, and then repeat with the figure-eight, doing upward circling movements. Make an effort to separate the toes at the beginning of each circling movement.

If you will follow out these ideas as well as the ideas on general care of the feet given later on in the chapter on Grooming, you should all your life be able to avoid reaching that awful moment when you have to admit that your feet are killing you.

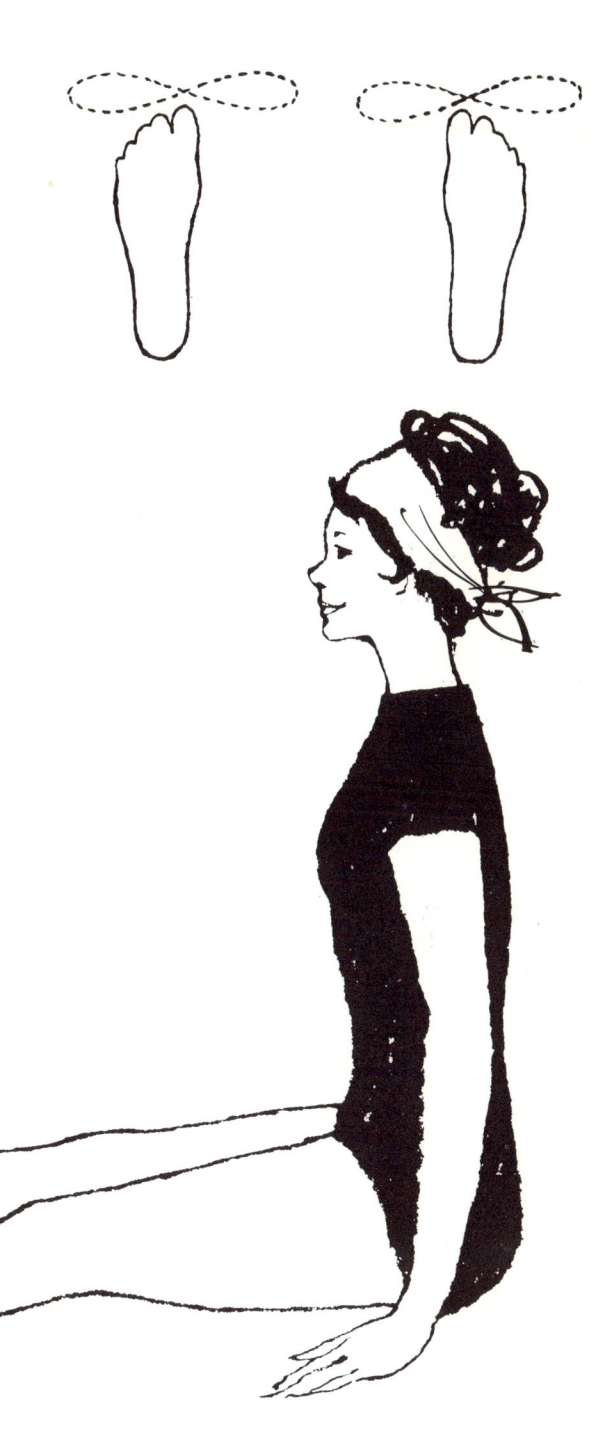

Figure standards

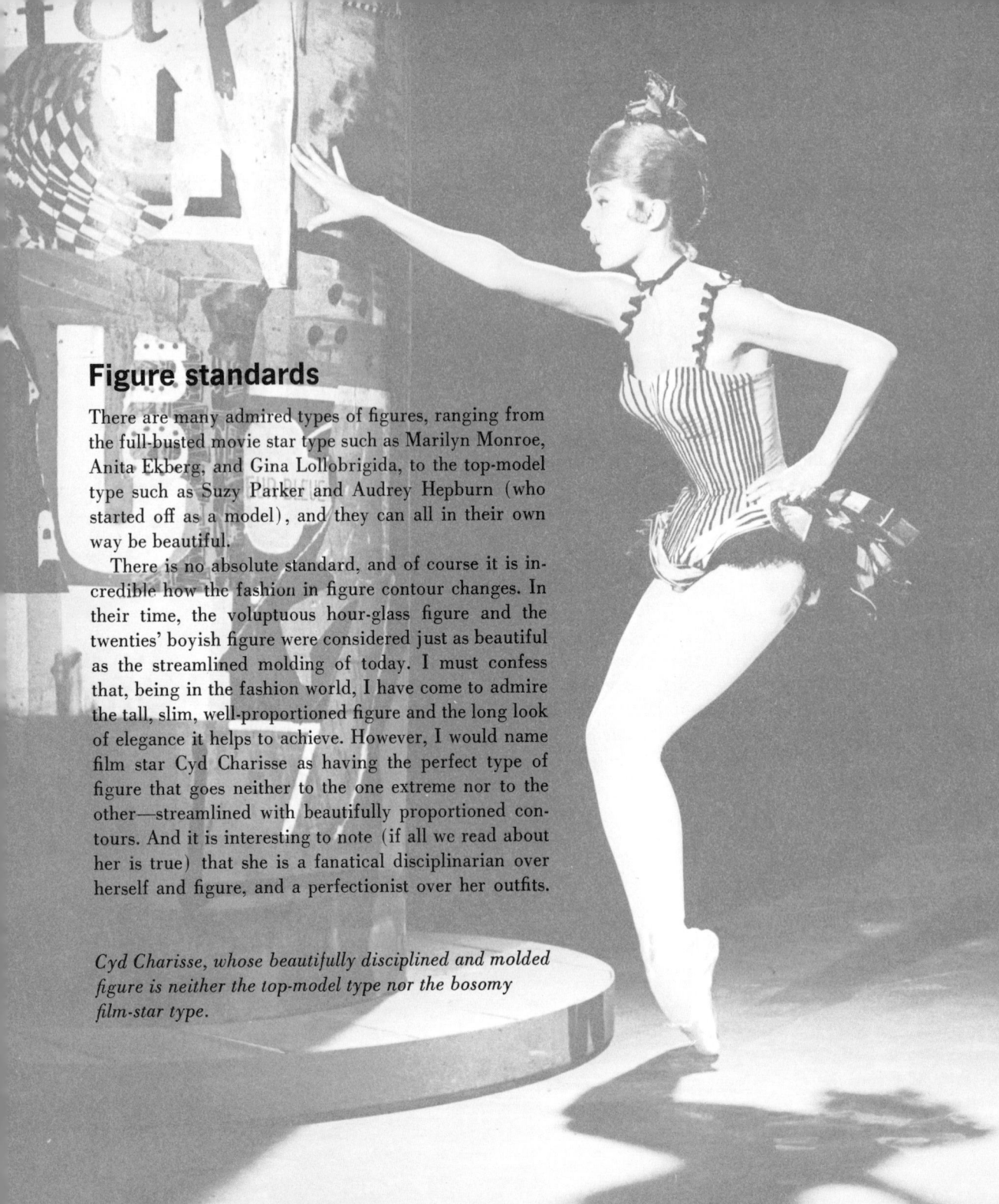

There are many admired types of figures, ranging from the full-busted movie star type such as Marilyn Monroe, Anita Ekberg, and Gina Lollobrigida, to the top-model type such as Suzy Parker and Audrey Hepburn (who started off as a model), and they can all in their own way be beautiful.

There is no absolute standard, and of course it is incredible how the fashion in figure contour changes. In their time, the voluptuous hour-glass figure and the twenties' boyish figure were considered just as beautiful as the streamlined molding of today. I must confess that, being in the fashion world, I have come to admire the tall, slim, well-proportioned figure and the long look of elegance it helps to achieve. However, I would name film star Cyd Charisse as having the perfect type of figure that goes neither to the one extreme nor to the other—streamlined with beautifully proportioned contours. And it is interesting to note (if all we read about her is true) that she is a fanatical disciplinarian over herself and figure, and a perfectionist over her outfits.

Cyd Charisse, whose beautifully disciplined and molded figure is neither the top-model type nor the bosomy film-star type.

5 makeup

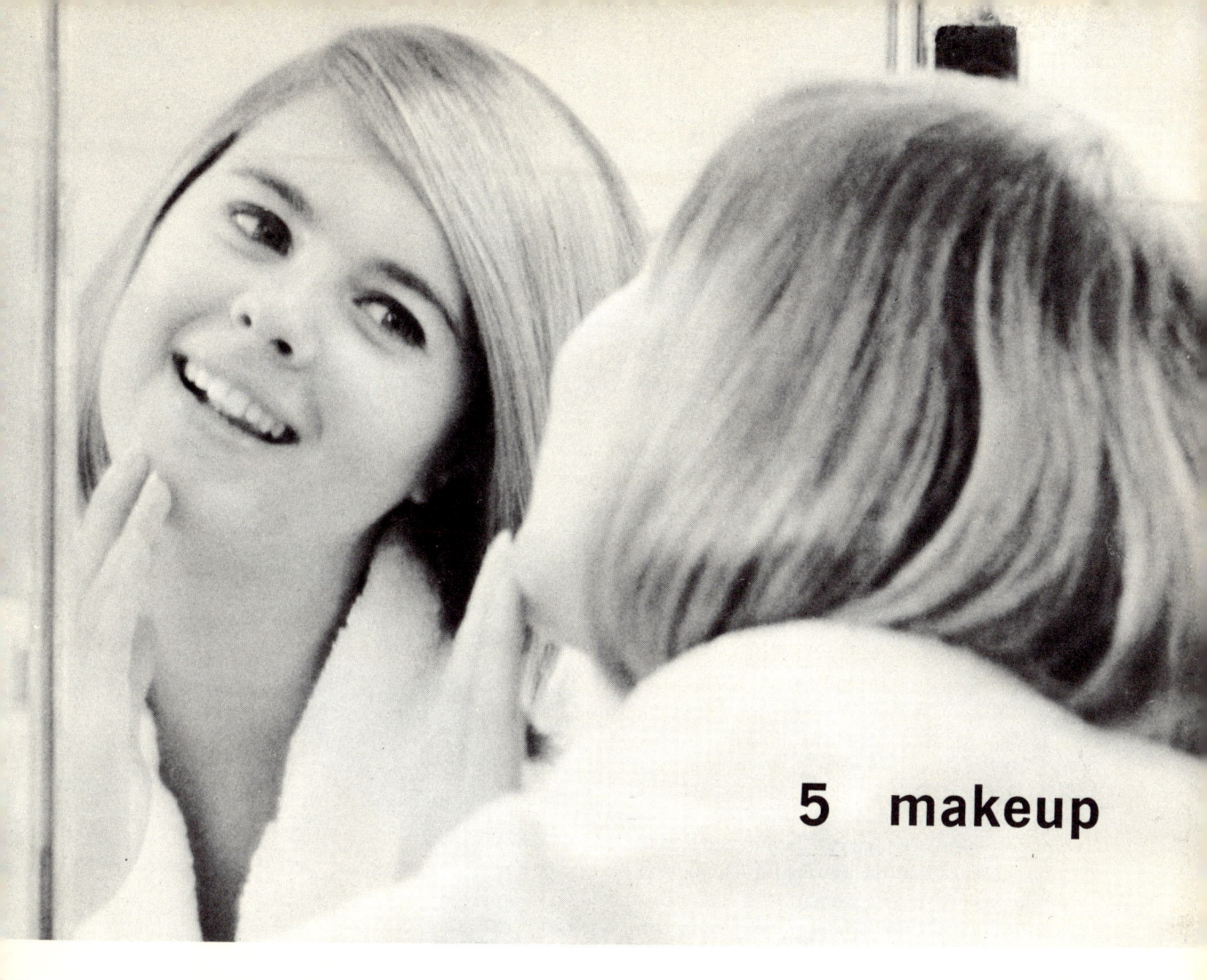

The sparing use of a pale lipstick is a suitable beginning when you first start to use makeup. Decide that from the very start you will always apply makeup neatly and professionally.

While you are acquiring your own skill, I suggest that you experiment with each detail of makeup until you yourself are satisfied with the result—thus in the sum total, something of your individuality emerges. Then later, when you *do* perhaps have a makeup at a beauty salon, while admiring the professional expertness you may well prefer your own version. This is as it should be!

Brands

At the beginning you are bound to wonder what brand of makeup to use. Here you have all my sympathy because there are so many good brands on the market (with fascinating new ones coming along from time to time) that it is quite bewildering for the beginner to know which will be the best for her. However, try buying small trial sizes where possible and experiment with the various shades considered right for your complexion and coloring. Don't buy a lot of cosmetics until you have tried a few different kinds and can, therefore, begin to form your opinion.

Equipment

Here are a few items you need for the professional approach:

A MAKEUP CAPE. This is to protect your clothes. (The cape should also be worn when you dress your hair.)

A HEAD BAND. One yard of elastic bandage about three inches wide is suitable. Tie it round your forehead, the knot in the nape of the neck, and then slide it up the forehead to the hairline. This will prevent hair falling over the face.

COTTON BATTING

PAPER TISSUES

BRUSHES (for lips, eye shadow, mascara)

CLOTHES BRUSH. For light carrying, the small nylon variety is best.

Complexion care

The continual use of makeup is not bad for the complexion provided that the routine for complexion care is faithfully observed. The woman who has used makeup all her life, but with scrupulous complexion care, often reaches the age of sixty or so with a better complexion than the woman of the same age who has never used makeup, and who has taken her complexion for granted and never bothered to give it any special care.

The magic routine is:

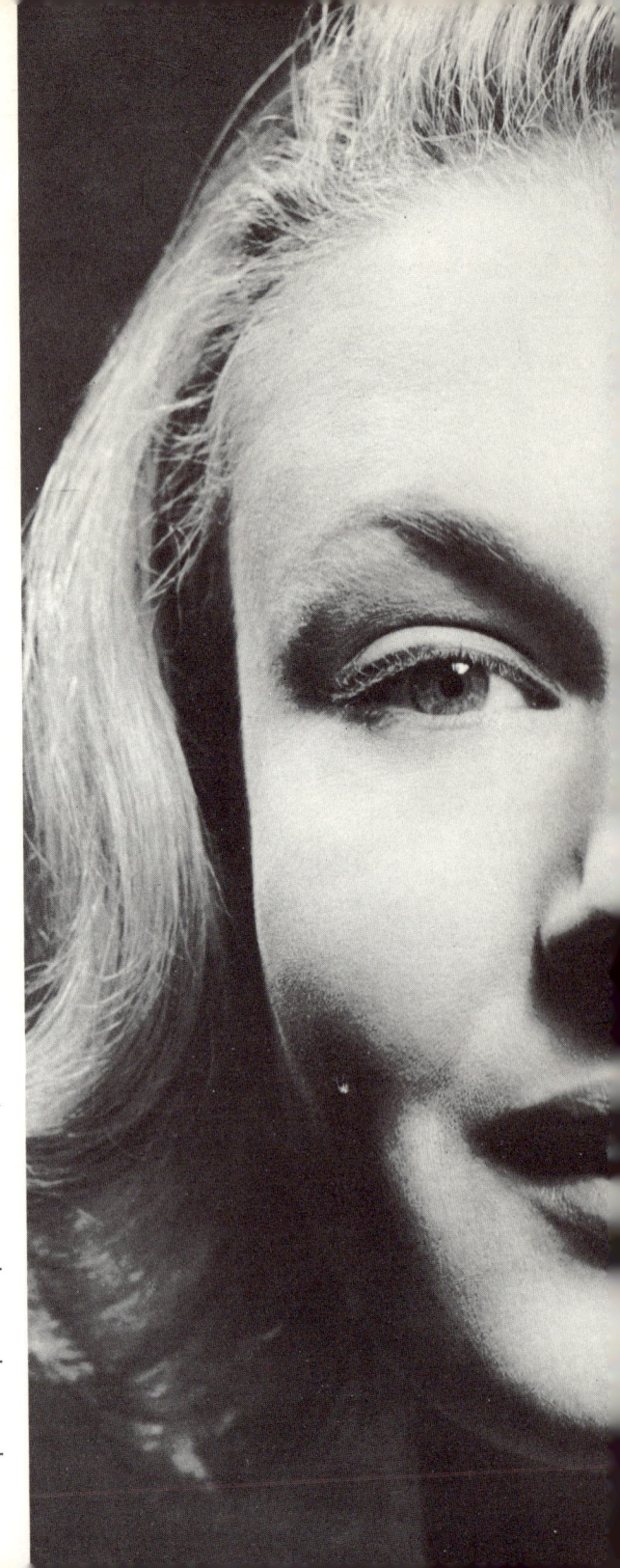

Cleanse

Tone

Nourish

cleanse

Here the great decision is to wash or not to wash. The important thing, however, is that the complexion should be really and thoroughly clean. If there has been only a light makeup, then warm water and a good mild soap will do the job. But a heavy makeup needs removing by the use of a cleansing cream or lotion. Should the skin tend to be dry, or adversely affected by, say, unaccustomed hard water, then there is a good cause for sticking to cleansing creams and lotions.

tone

(a) Cold water—when you splash your face with cold water—or pat it gently with cotton batting wrung out in cold water—the pores close, and you are toning the complexion.

(b) Skin tonics, toning lotions—these do the same thing, but they are perhaps a little more exciting to use than cold water.

(c) Astringents—these do the job too, but are stronger than tonics and toning lotions. It is best to use them only sparingly.

nourish

This means the application of a skin food. Be sure to get the correct one for your skin, normal, dry, or greasy.

the times for the routine

The most important time is before going to bed. As a matter of fact, one of the quickest ways in which to ruin the complexion is to go to bed with makeup on. The body warmth gathering round you while you sleep will cause the pores to open and then the stale makeup plus the dust of the day will tend to sink in. If you have ever gone to bed lazily without cleansing off the makeup and then looked at the state of your complexion in the morning, you will know what I mean. For similar reasons, the routine should be carried out before a bath.

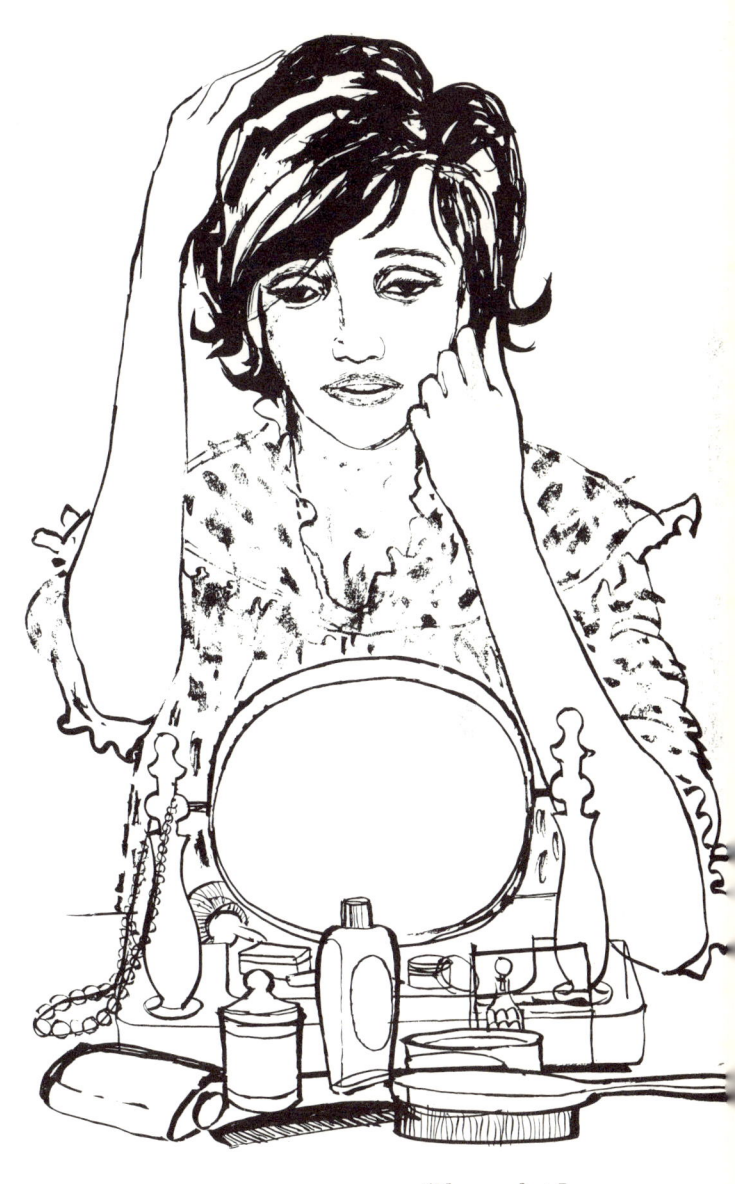

. . . you will know what I mean

The order of making up

Let us suppose you are making up first thing in the morning.

Cleanse however efficiently you cleansed at night, a thorough cleansing is still required in the morning.

Tone and *tone and tone*, in order to get the complexion smooth and cold. This gets you off to a good start because if the complexion is hot, the makeup is probably spoiling even while you are applying it.

Foundation this should be applied sparingly and thoroughly over the whole of the complexion including the eyelids and just beyond the jawline. Be sure the foundation matches the skin of the neck. Nothing looks more peculiar than being confronted with a milk-and-roses complexion above a brownish neck or a would-be sun-tanned look above a milky white neck. If your complexion tends to be dry, apply a moisturizer or a little skin food before the foundation. This is a good tip anyway because a foundation will always go on more smoothly and evenly if the complexion has been rendered a little tacky.

Cream Rouge (*if used*) don't use rouge unless you look absolutely ill without it. An obviously rouged look has been out of date for a long time. But if you must use it, try applying it in a T formation over the cheek bone, and then merge it well in.

Eye Shadow (*if used*) experiment as to *where* you place it (perhaps covering about half the lid, or keeping it to a narrow line and bringing it out high and wide), but in any case let the color come right to the edge of the lid. If you leave a gap of uncovered lid between the shadow and the edge of the lid, you lose the look of glamour you are trying to build up. Eye shadow can also be applied more as a line on the lid edge (absolutely meeting the mascara on the lashes) and this can quite successfully be done after powdering.

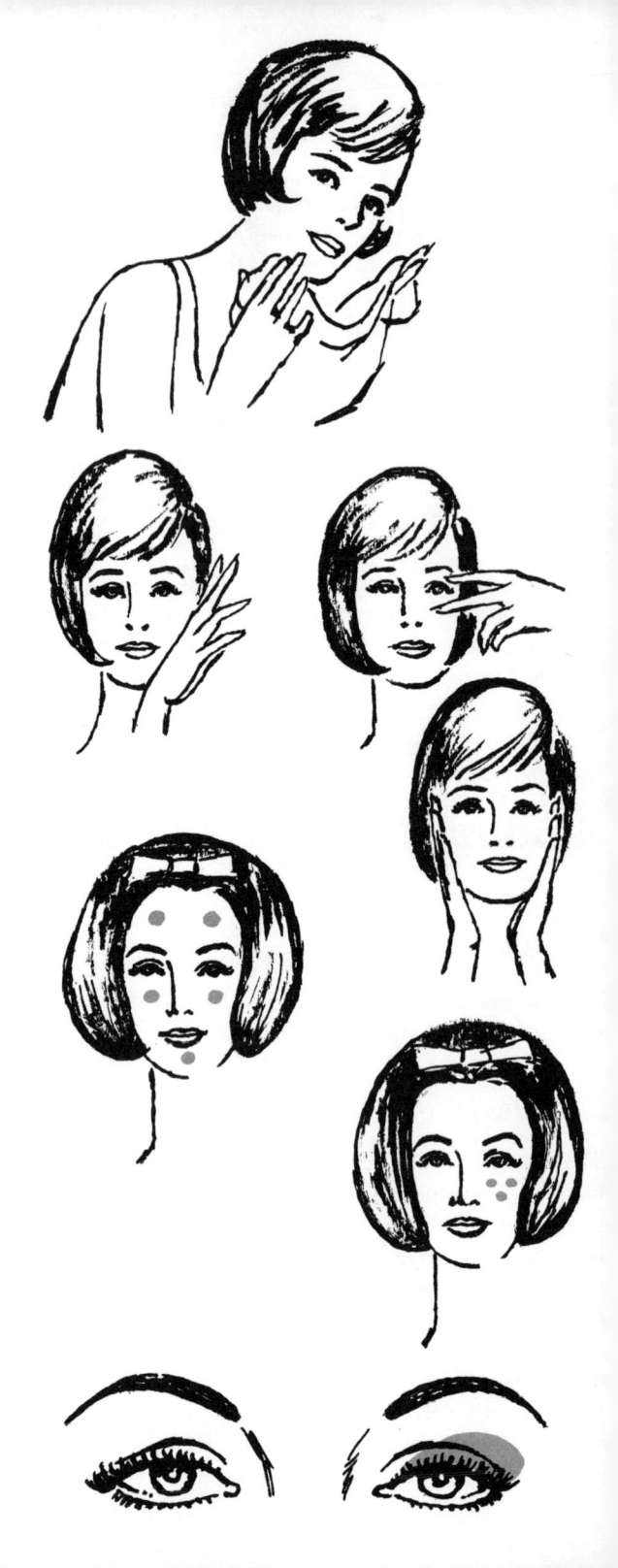

Powder use this generously over the whole face. Loose powder keeps fresher looking, but cake powder is useful for giving the makeup a final lasting finish. Keep two shades of powder, one a little deeper than the other, so that you can keep pace with slight changes of skin tone.

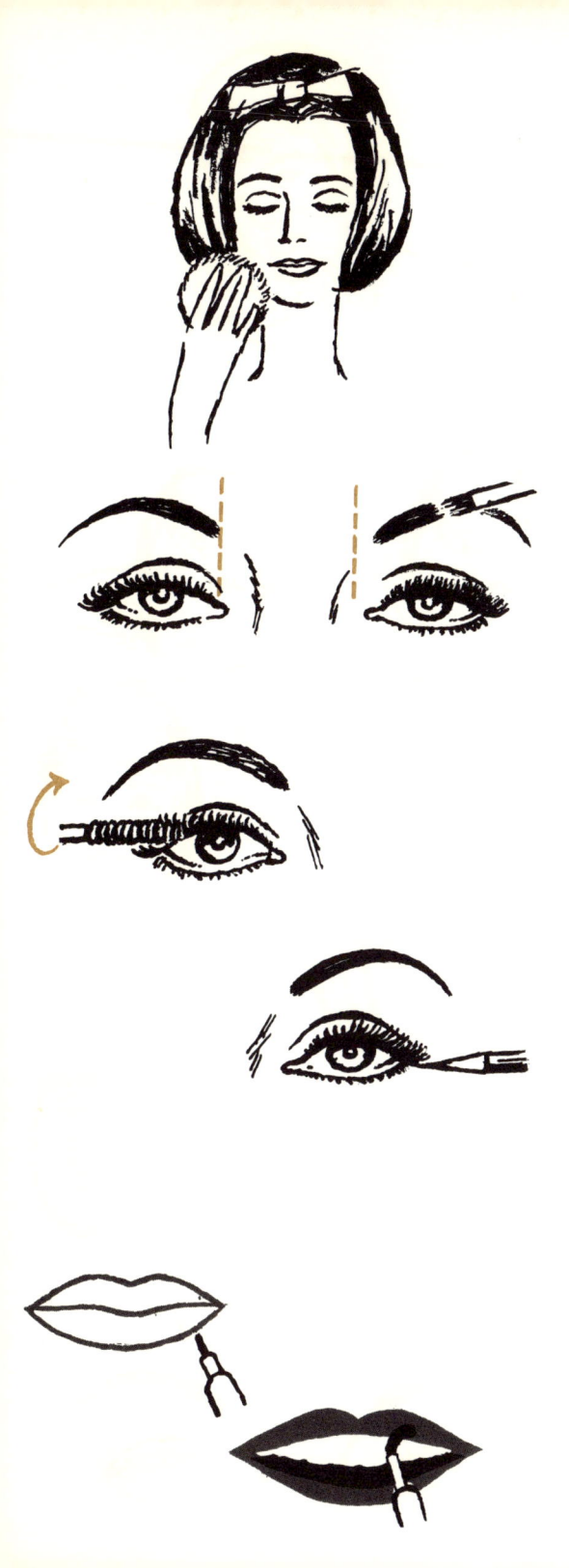

Eyebrows first brush any powder out of the brows (a clean leftover mascara brush is good for this). At the same time, brush the brows into their best shape. If they are a little colorless, then later on you could apply sparingly a little mascara—probably the amount left on your brush after attending to lashes will be sufficient. Examine the shape of the brows generally. For a wide-eyed look, they should be a little farther apart than are the eyes. If you decide to trim them up a little (with a good pair of tweezers) then be sure to study first the nose to eyebrow contour—and aim to get the eyebrows looking as though they naturally followed the bone contour of the nose.

Mascara this can be used for the lashes, the eyebrows, and eyelines. Brush lashes outwards—coaxing as many as possible to the outer corners. Brush *both sides* (top and underneath) of the upper lashes. Put mascara on the lower lashes only if, after you have tried it as an experiment, you find this suits you.

Eyebrow pencil this can be used for shaping the eyebrows and for drawing eyelines. These lines—to achieve their glamorous purpose—must be on the very edge of the lid and meet the mascara on the lashes. To work efficiently the pencil needs frequent sharpening. Use a razor blade in a holder to sharpen the end to a chisel edge.

The mouth persevere with the use of the lip brush. Once you have mastered the art, you will see how much more groomed the mouth looks. Work the brush on the lipstick much as you would a brush on paint, at the same time guiding the brush to a chisel-shaped edge. Hold this chisel edge at right angles to the edge of the lips and outline the whole mouth. Follow by blocking in—brushing and brushing and brushing. The more you brush the lipstick in, the longer the mouth will remain groomed.

12 makeup tips

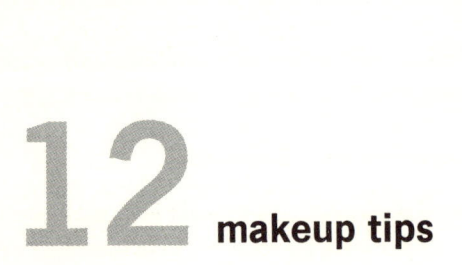

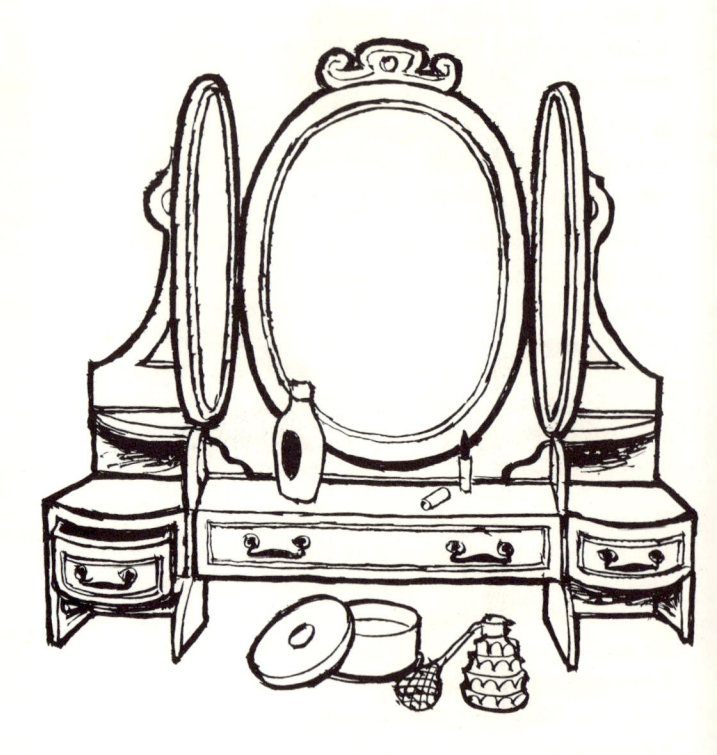

1 LOOKING GLASS—the one at your dressing table should have its back to the light. Your hand mirror should be in frequent use for close inspection. A magnifying mirror can be a great help if your eyesight is poor.

2 TREASURE YOUR COMPLEXION—it is the only one you will ever have. Whatever the operation, use the fingers on it only lightly, allowing them to skate over the surface of the skin rather than exert any pressure. Whenever possible, use swirling, upward, massagelike movements. When using a washcloth or hand towel on the face, just work and pat; do not rub and pull.

3 ALL-PURPOSE SKIN CREAMS—if you use these, then keep the operation of cleansing quite separate from the operation of nourishing. In any case the toning should come between the two.

4 ROUND THE EYES—use all makeup sparingly in this area. You can easily get a dried-up look.

5 FACIAL CONTOURS—learn to appreciate these as would a sculptor. They can have unsuspected beauty of their own.

6 OVERFULL LIPS—apply foundation and powder over the whole mouth, and then underplay the lipline when applying the lipstick.

7 ROSEBUD MOUTH—this was at one time the fashionable mouth, but is so no longer. Overplay the lipline when applying the lipstick. Of course, the mouth can only be overplayed vertically, not horizontally. Merely increase the width of the curve of the top or lower lip (or of both). However, before doing this, make sure that the space between top lip and nose, or between bottom lip and chin, is enough to allow it.

8 HIGH FOREHEAD—this may look perfectly all right, but if you're not satisfied with the way it looks, try the effect of reducing the distance between the eyes and the hairline by increasing the upward curve of the eyebrows (using the eyebrow pencil). If the hairline and brow already suggest a roundness, then avoid a repetition of roundness in the eyebrow by penciling them up a fraction at the outer corners.

9 BROAD JAW—a darker foundation blended carefully over the jawline helps to fade it out and it becomes far less noticeable.

10 LARGE FACE—this can be given an illusion of looking smaller by applying either a darker foundation or a delicate shading of cream rouge, down the sides of the cheeks.

11 NOSE IN WINTER—if it gets pink, then use enough rouge to keep the cheeks a little pinker than the nose.

12 NOSE IN SUMMER—if this tends to become overbrown or overpink from the sun, then protect it rather specially with suntan cream or foundation, and again, use enough rouge to keep the cheeks a little pinker than the nose.

some general advice

In deciding how much makeup to use, be guided by what is suitable for the occasion, the season and the time of day. On vacation, for instance, while maintaining eye, eyebrow, and mouth makeup, it is a good plan to abandon normal foundation and powder and use only a good suntan cream, which can be reapplied from time to time. This may be particularly desirable if you are out for hours in hot sunshine.

If anything could be labeled a gimmick (such as green eyelashes, black lipstick), then it is only suitable for a fancy-dress party—and out of place for general social occasions or for business.

If you don't really care for makeup at all, then use just enough to give you a groomed look, get rid of highlights, shines or a too high color.

6 dress

General principles

Do you realize that in the sum total of your appearance *one* wrong or uncared-for item can ruin the whole? Behind this simple question lies one broad general aim for the well-dressed young woman—*the clothes, the accessories, and the grooming* must all be right in every detail. Imagine the picture of the girl whose clothes, accessories, manicure, makeup are all nearly perfect, but the hair is lank and uncared-for; or if the hair is perfect, imagine the picture if she is wearing a pair of shabby, brown oxfords with an otherwise impeccable navy-and-white ensemble.

Do you realize that even if you're wearing a marvelous outfit, you're not a well-dressed young woman if it isn't *suitable for the occasion?* The hour, the day, the time of the year, the place, and the occasion should all be considered in choosing the outfit to be worn. Imagine a girl turning up for work at 9 A.M. wearing a really smashing low-cut cocktail dress, or for a friend's party in a glorious ski outfit.

When you get an unexpected invitation, do you find you have nothing to wear? This is indeed bad planning. You should learn to assess the overall dress demands of your life, and build up a wardrobe to meet them. This is another broad principle upon which to work.

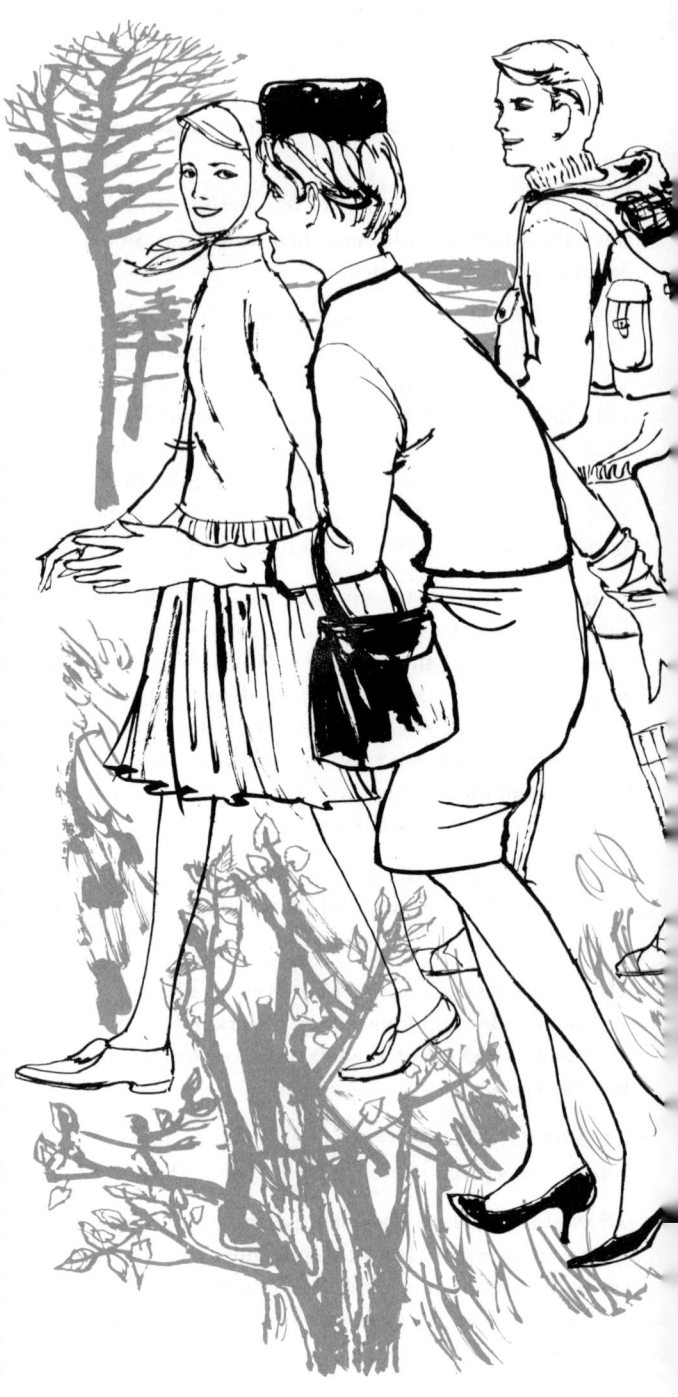

Do you hate all your clothes? You lose harmony if you have pushed yourself into styles which your own artistic sense says are ugly (despite the fact that they may be high fashion). You lose harmony if you do not like the color of your outfit. And you lose harmony if you can't bear the feel of the material of your outfit. But probably the basic reason you are dissatisfied is that you have never really given enough thought to the subject of dress, nor realized that it is one of the most delightfully feminine means of expressing your individuality.

Developing a dress sense

Rid your mind of the idea that you will automatically develop a dress sense as you grow older. Tune in now to fashion trends and the golden rules of dress by deliberate study along the following general lines.

By regular scrutiny of leading fashion magazines. These are often available at your library, or you could share the expense with a friend. As you turn the pages, allow the eye and mind to absorb proportions, general line, neckline, lengths, sleeves, accessories, costume jewelry, hair styles, and above all the uncluttered look of the models in the pictures.

By reading avidly the fashion articles and the woman's page in your family newspapers. This can be particularly rewarding when the fashion journalists are reporting on their visits to see new styles and new collections. Many of the women journalists have been studying and writing about fashion all their lives, and their considered, wise, and often witty comments on what they see can guide you in acquiring your own sense of fashion value.

By keeping an open mind about how you will apply your growing new knowledge. Some of your old loves may be right for you, and some of the new ideas quite wrong, and vice versa. Only when you have the overall picture of rules and trends can you unerringly and confidently sort out not only what is right for your figure and general physical appearance, but what will also be in harmony with your personality (whether demure or one with a streak of showmanship).

By having critical dress sessions in the privacy of your room in front of your full-length looking glass. Your looking glass should, of course, be placed back to a window, and it is essential to work in cold, hard daylight. Artificial lighting or sunlight can cast glamorous shadows over your reflection and may prevent you from reaching the clear assessment you are seeking.

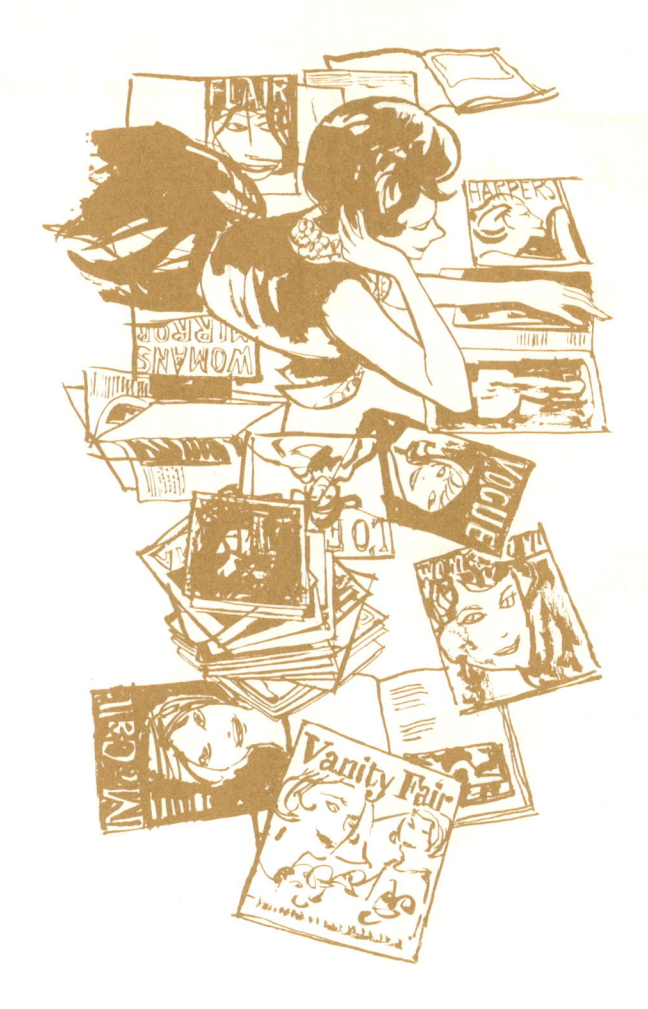

This time and hard work spent over your effects in private is neither a sign of conceit nor wasted. The whole object is eventually to be able to meet your world with such supreme confidence in your appearance that you can forget it—and so be able to concentrate upon what are, after all, the more important things of life, your family, your friends, your leisure activities, and above all, your career. Let us here face it fairly and squarely, that we women feel self-conscious all the time if we are not satisfied with our appearance. This can result in loss of self-confidence and concentration.

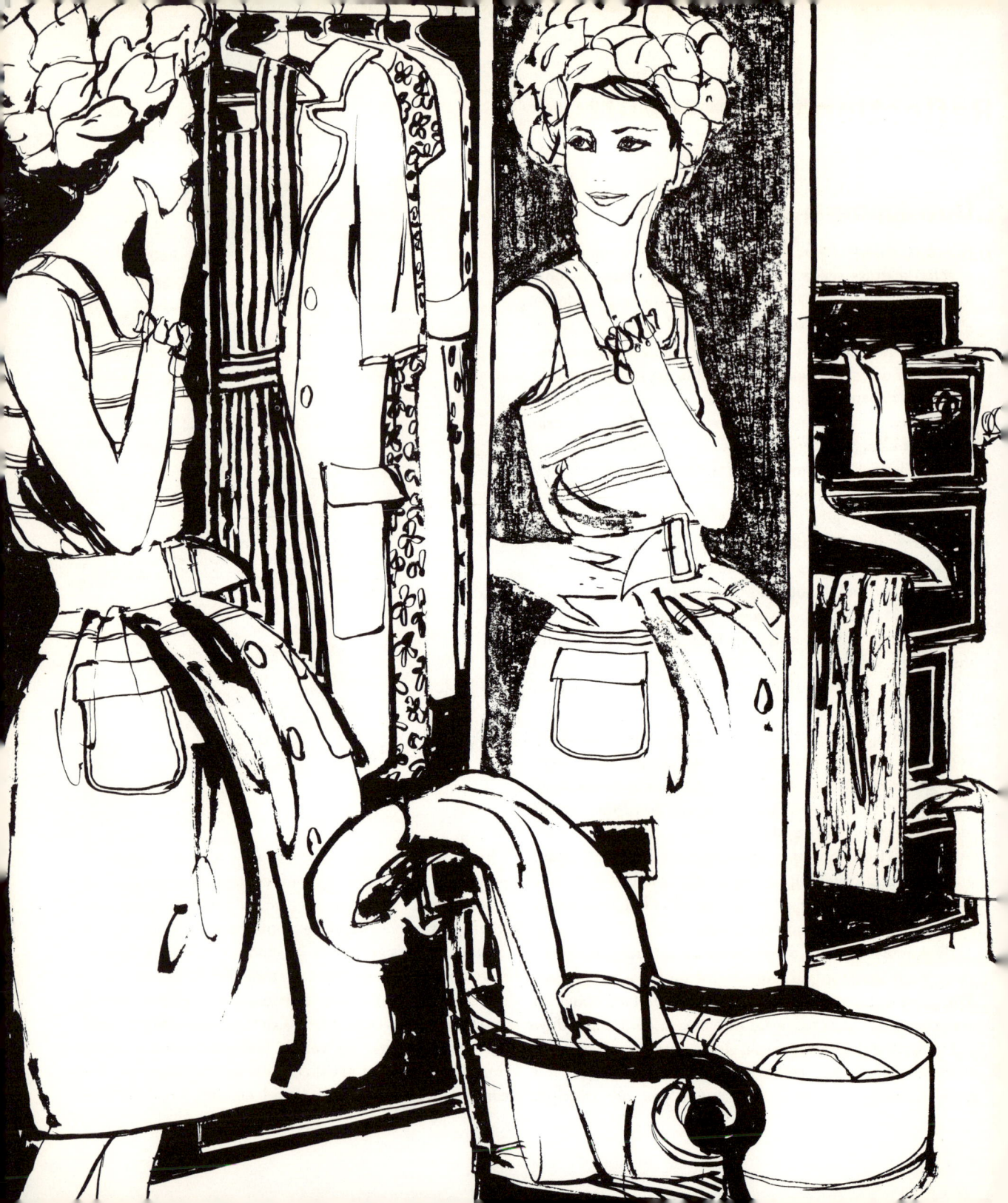

Reflections in the Mirror

Here are some of the questions, queries, and comments to hurl at your reflection in the mirror.

Does the overall effect look right?

If the answer is "no," then a systematic analysis of lengths, line, accessories, etc., should be made. If faults can't be remedied, or if the outfit just isn't right for your figure, then if possible discard the outfit rather than make yourself miserable by trying to get your wear out of it.

Does the general line and impression satisfy me?

Your *own* preferences and sense of beauty and line must take over here. Have you perhaps blindly pushed yourself into the latest fashion without thought as to whether you like it or not, and whether it suits you?

Do I look cluttered?

It is impossible to look well turned out with that essential air of casual simplicity if there are too many items making up the whole. Items must include buttons, belts, buckles, trimmings, any special features, scarves, bows, all costume jewelry, glasses, visible pins, clips, combs in the hair, handbags, shoes, gloves. Since shoes, gloves, handbags, glasses are probably among your essentials, then you begin to see how restrained you must be about the rest. You may discover that you appear cluttered by what you have added to an outfit, and, therefore, this can be remedied. If, however, you discover that the outfit is inherently cluttered before you have added any accessories, then you have learned a valuable lesson and a basic one. Most of your clothes should look starkly simple before the addition of accessories. This will in future guide you when shopping, and you will not be misled by gimmicks or special features and special contrasts, etc.

If eyeglasses are a must, then accept them as one of your accessories and take special care in choosing the shape, size, and color of the frames. Try on empty frames until you find the right one for you. You may find it best to choose a color that harmonizes with your hair, eyebrows, eyes, or basic color scheme. On the other hand you may find that the biggest, blackest frames you can find simply emphasize your femininity by sheer contrast. There are many experts to guide you over this. I know a woman with years of experience in both the world of fashion *and* of optics who knows that many girls suffer a sense of inferiority because of the necessity to wear spectacles, and in many cases where she has given her help in the selection of frames she has been thrilled to notice the good psychological effect on a girl when the expertly chosen frames are seen to complement the appearance or add interest, rather than the reverse.

How many colors am I wearing?

One of fashion's golden rules is "never more than three." (This, of course, doesn't apply when you are wearing specially patterned materials, such as a paisley pattern which is in itself multicolored.)

Do I look "musical comedy"?

In other words, are you decked out in strong, gay color contrasts? If you find you're wearing red, white, and blue, or the three colors of a national flag, then this is awful. As a matter of fact, as your dress sense develops, you will probably discover for yourself that obvious color contrasts, such as purple/yellow, blue/red, yellow/blue, and green/yellow lack subtlety when applied to dress. If your outfit is in a color, it is best to go for matching accessories or black and white.

Do my separates part in the middle?

This is very bad dressing, particularly if a bare midriff is revealed. Care should be taken to see that blouse and skirt stay trimly together at the waistline.

Do I look "big" or "square"?

Perhaps thick material is giving you unwanted bulk all over. Perhaps a flared skirt is accentuating width at the hip or seat. Perhaps a set-in sleeve is accentuating shoulders which are already on the broad side. Or perhaps the sleeves themselves are too wide. Should you be looking particularly big between waist and thigh, then perhaps you're ruining your line with too many petticoats.

Do I look "plastered"?

No, I don't mean, do you look a little "tight", but have you put on too many white or pastel accessories? For instance, white hat, collar, cuffs, belt, shoes, and handbag with a black or navy outfit is just too much. *One* white accessory can look superb, *two* nice, *three or more* begin to give you the "plastered" look. Accessories that match one's outfit are always nice. Black shoes and a black handbag go with nearly everything.

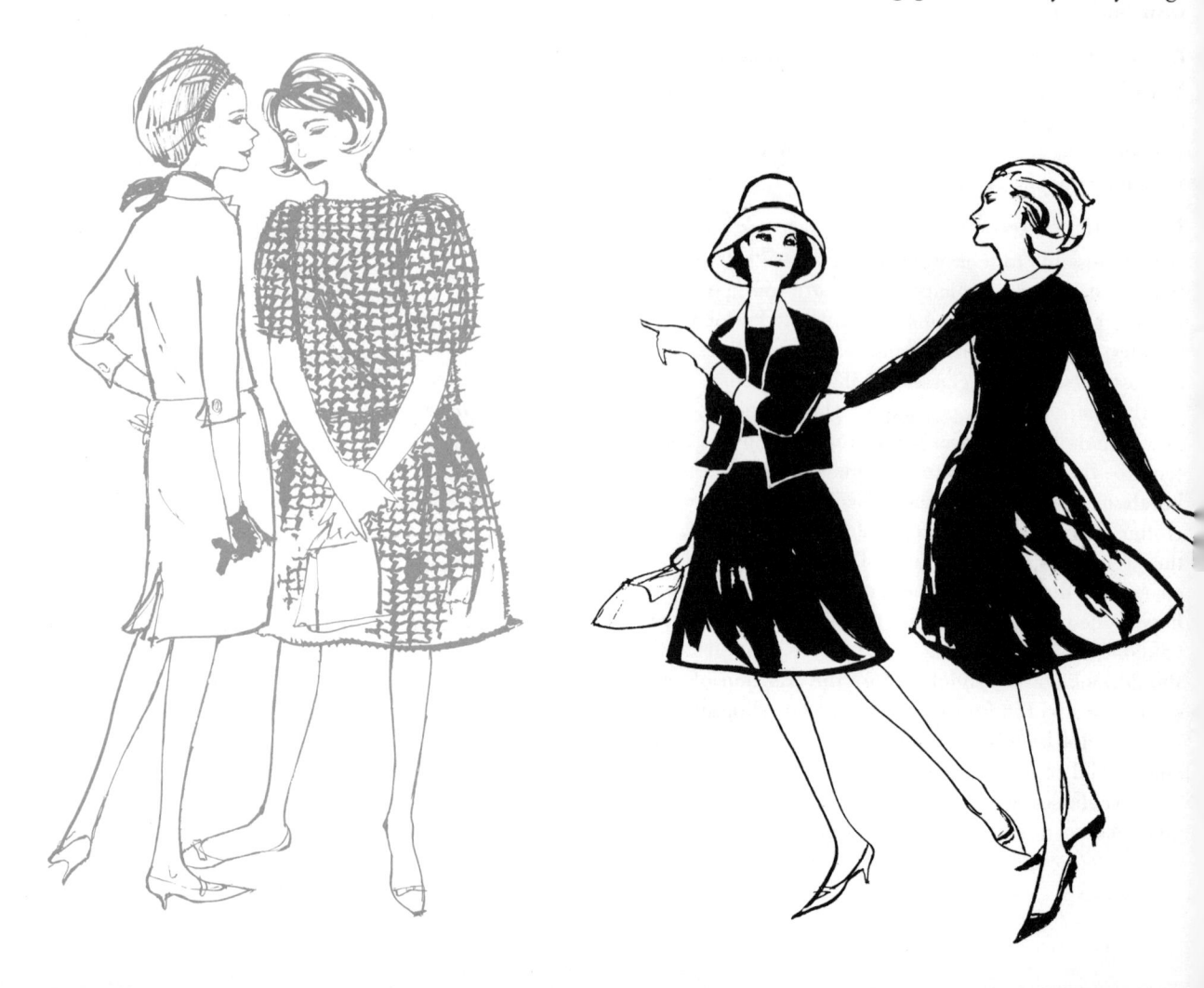

Do I look pear-shaped?

You may in fact be basically pear-shaped, (small bust, wide hips—many women are like this); but you may have chosen outfits which accentuate this instead of disguising it. It may be that the top is slim and trim and the skirt bulky. Obviously you should reverse this, and your best line is probably either to wear a bolero-length top or one that reaches the hips; but not a top which seems to rest on your widest part. A good bra with built-in accentuation or good uplift will help to give a fuller look. If you're short as well as pear-shaped, then choose lines with a waist, or with a waist indicated.

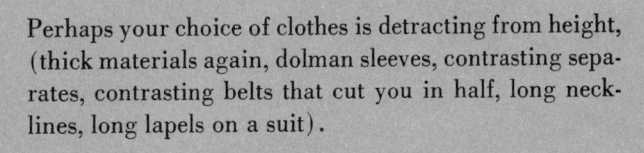

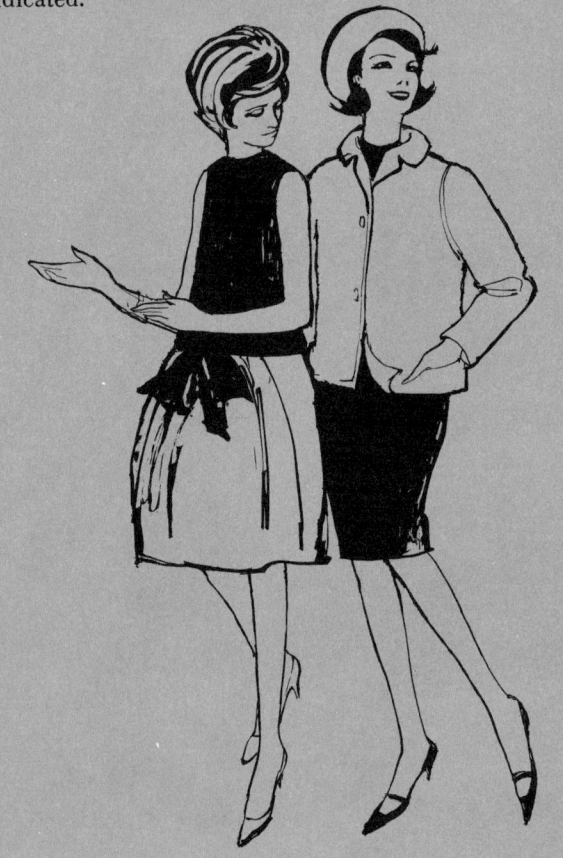

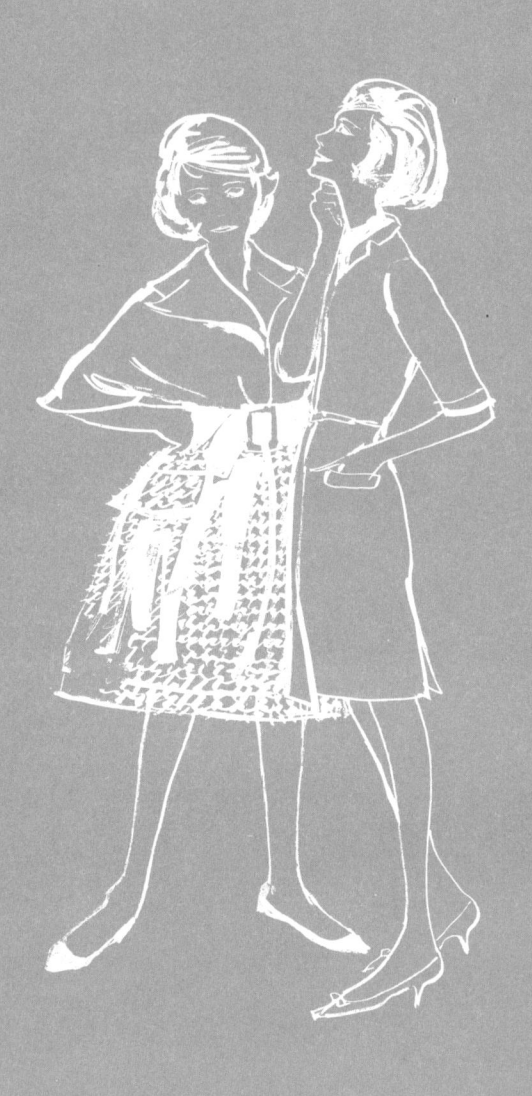

Do I look unnecessarily short?

Perhaps your choice of clothes is detracting from height, (thick materials again, dolman sleeves, contrasting separates, contrasting belts that cut you in half, long necklines, long lapels on a suit).

My neck looks frightfully long!

Wonderful. Apart from a long body, nothing will give you the look of a model better than a long neckline, provided you let the neck show and don't clutter it up.

I don't seem to have much neck!

Maybe your neck *is* short. But are you tending to let it disappear by drowning it in too-long hair, standup collars, and costume jewelry?

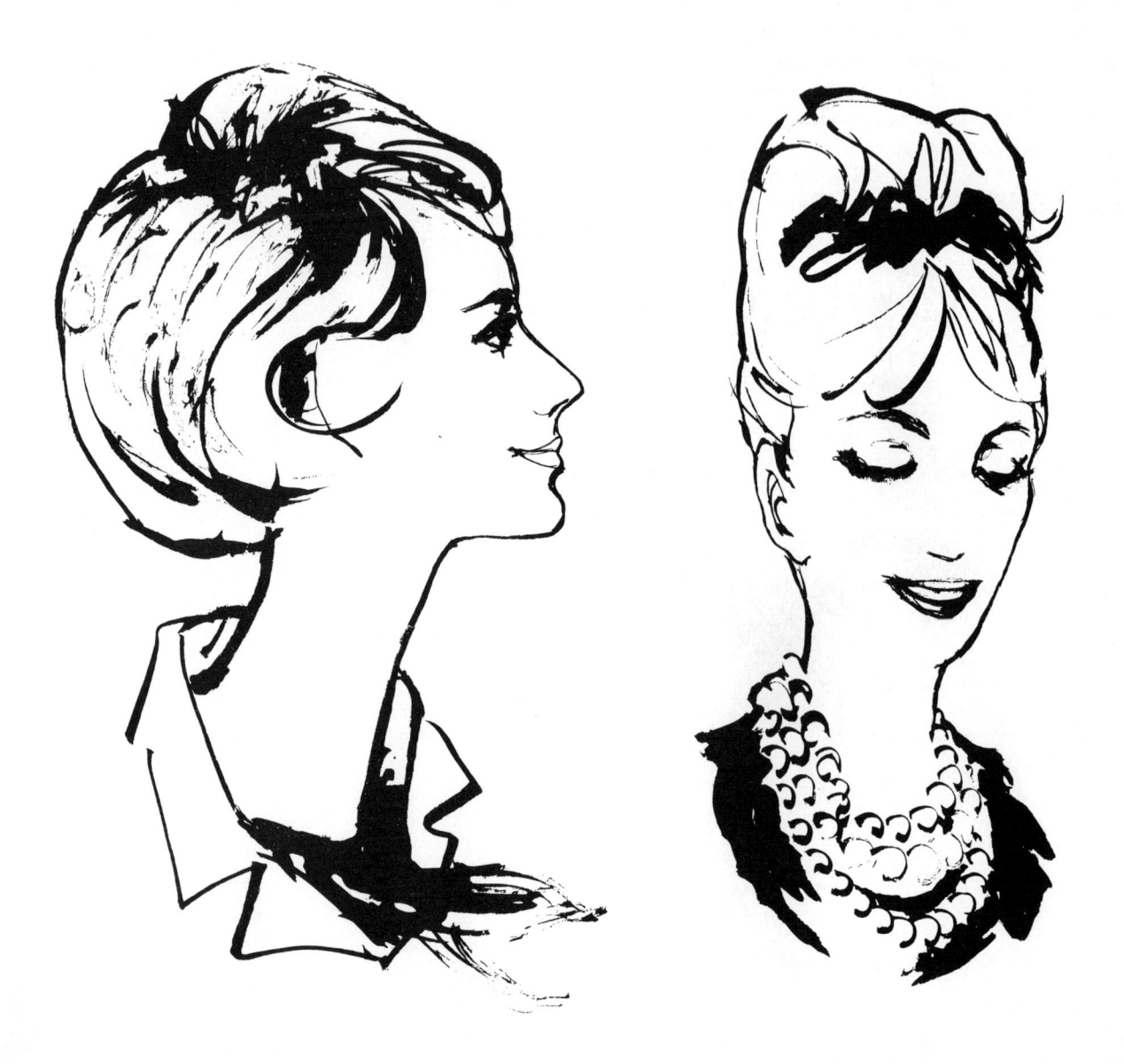

Are my necklines right?

If everything about you is pretty normal and well-proportioned, then you can probably wear any line that you fancy. If you have sloping or narrow shoulders, a small collarless neckline should look right—and preferably with at least a small sleeve. (A wide neckline takes up too much of your width and a sleeveless garment can give you a chopped-off, narrow look.) For evening, a bare top, or an off-the-shoulder neckline should be the most flattering. Broad shoulders can take a wide or scooped out neckline, and sleeveless garments too. A broad jaw looks best framed by a neckline that is a little wider than itself. All this is only very general guidance. I'm only too well aware that some people have narrow shoulders, a broad jaw, *and* a short neck to cope with, and if so, then care must be taken until the best line has been found.

Are my gloves the right length?

A teenager can get away with short gloves with almost anything, but the general rule is that the shorter the sleeve, the longer the glove. With a sleeveless day dress, the glove which reaches the elbow is best (not worn pulled up straight, but pushed down a little). With full evening dress, the gloves should reach above the elbow. Avoid prettied-up gloves. When wearing matching gloves, avoid the animal-paw look by allowing a space for the bare arm to show between glove and sleeve. Gloves should always be worn with a hat; they can be carried when you are without a hat or otherwise informally dressed. Full-length gloves should not be worn with a day or cocktail dress with sleeves.

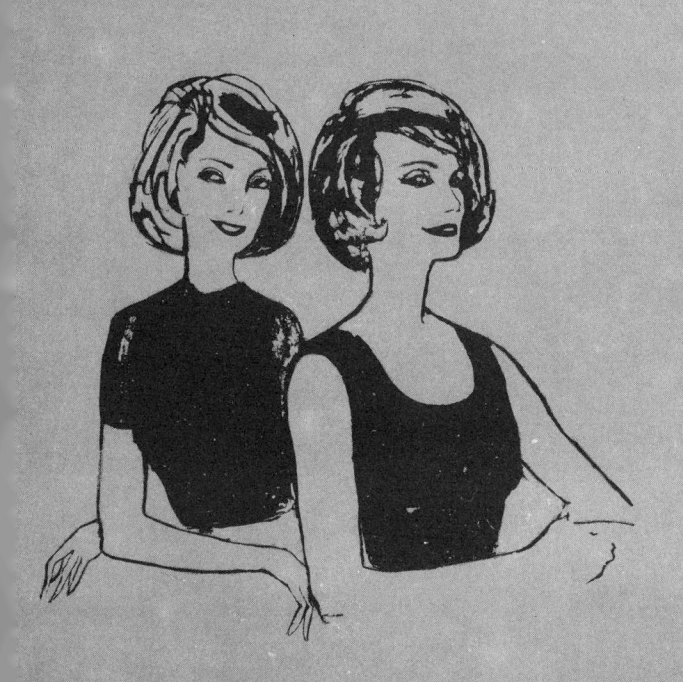

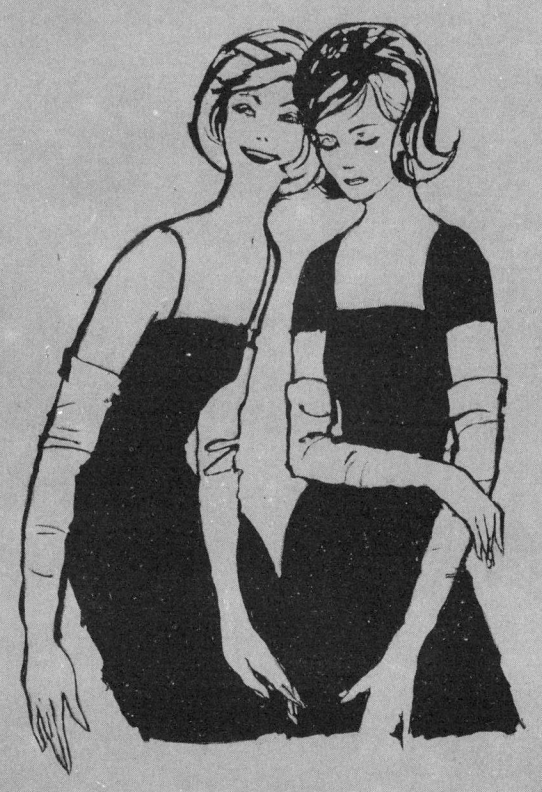

I think I look frightful in hats!

We all go through this stage, but most of us gradually come to appreciate the intriguing versatility in looks that hats can provide. Either a hat should be that utterly simple thing that just rounds off your appearance, or it should be that creation that really does something for you or that is fabulous. Have you ever tried the combination of upswept hair (long or short), small simple hat with a matching veil that goes over the whole head? The effect is elegant and bewitching. *But get your hair right before you embark on hats.*

Are my stockings the right shade for my outfit?

All the natural flesh shades look right with most outfits. The darker or stronger shades may not look right with light outfits. The trend for very dark or black stockings comes and goes.

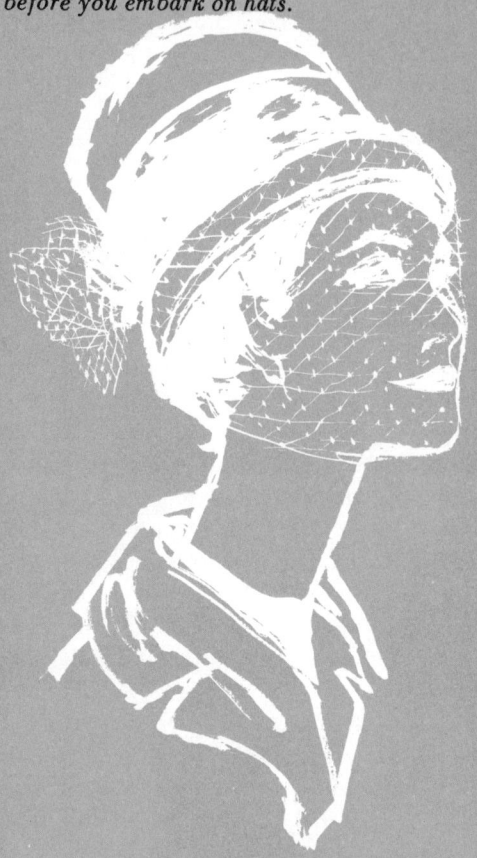

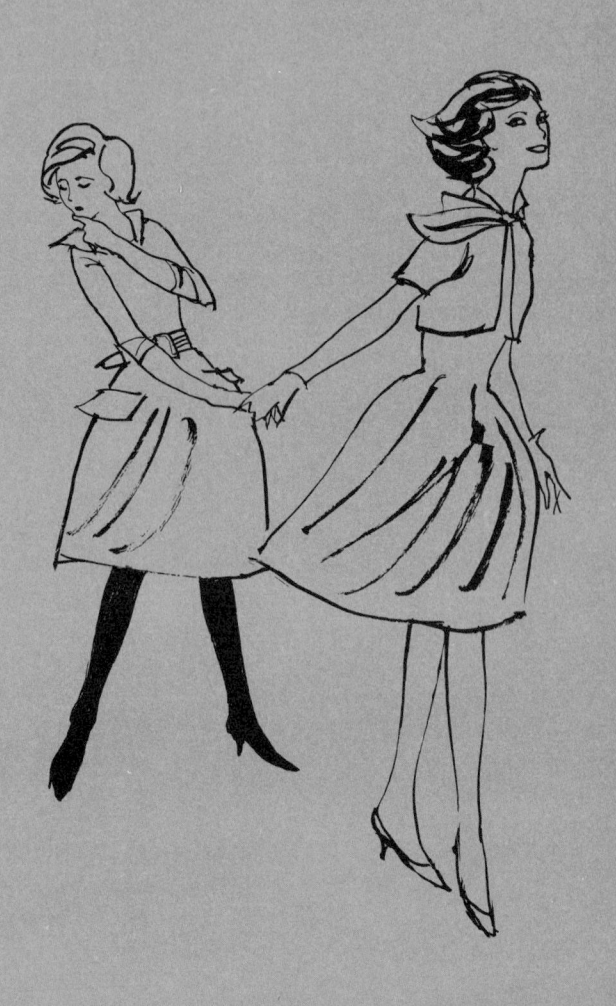

Building up your wardrobe

Reorganize your existing wardrobe, and while you are putting it in apple-pie order, set aside for only casual wear garments which don't conform to your growing dress sense.

Consider the nucleus that *is* satisfactory, and see if there is any basic scheme or color here on which you can build.

After you have decided what your own best color is then build your wardrobe around it so everything you have will go together. Of course, consider the colors that suit your skin, eyes, and hair, as well as the colors that appeal to you. No one can really decide this question of color *for* you, particularly as it can be quite a personal psychological problem. Friends may tell you that you look marvelous in, say, brown, but perhaps you had to wear a brown school uniform for ten years or so, and *you* feel you never want to wear the color again as long as you live.

Decide where there are gaps in your wardrobe (a suit, a coat, or a day dress?), and make a list of your needs in strict order of priority.

Shopping

Before you actually buy the garment at the top of your list, train yourself to be a good shopper. While you are doing this in the way I shall suggest, you will be testing out and improving your dress sense, and you will be getting an overall picture of the ways in which the fashion designers have translated the new trends and ideas which you have been following in your fashion study.

For a week or so pay as many visits as you can to the best stores that sell the garment you are seeking. Keep reminding yourself that you *are only looking around with no intention of buying.* Browse around the relevant departments, taking in styles, colors, tailoring, materials, and prices.

After a week or so of this, allow yourself to graduate to trying on garments. You need plenty of time to do this in order to feel unhurried and relaxed. Ask a lot of questions about the material, make, price of garment, and brood over your reflection in the looking glass (back, front, and sideways reflection, of course). When you are satisfied that the garment is for you, then buy it. If you feel it is wrong, thank the assistant and leave. When you have proceeded on these lines, you will be thankful you didn't buy the first thing that pleased you. During the looking you will probably have changed your mind many times about color and style, and you will certainly find that you are beginning to acquire a precious sense of reliability in your own dress sense and in your ability to handle shopping situations.

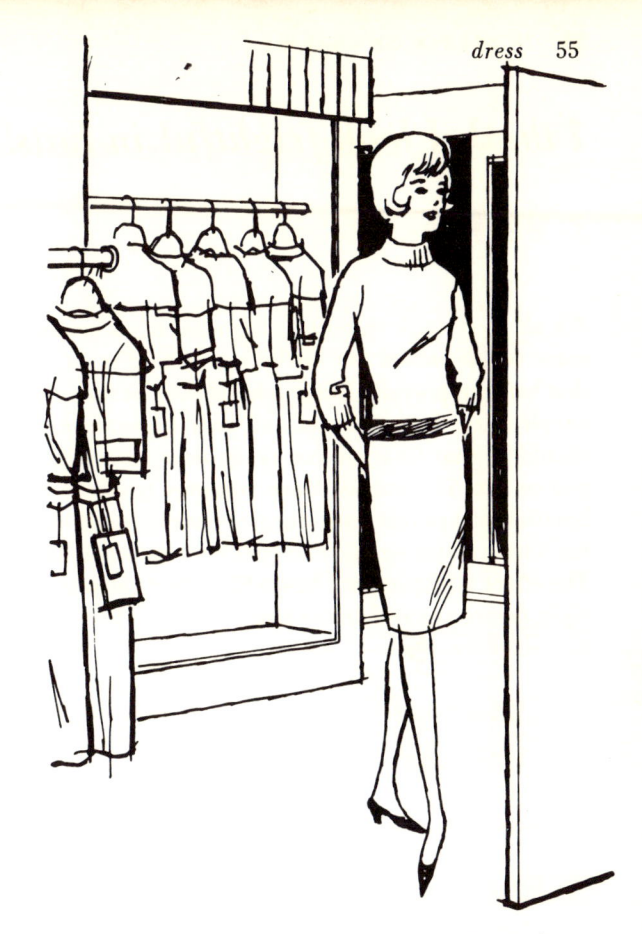

Each new item of your wardrobe should be selected with the utmost care. Be quite sure that it will take its place in your wardrobe along with the existing items, and be quite sure that you will love it from the very first moment until it is worn out.

The hard core of any young woman's wardrobe

1 Basic garments

Suits   Dresses
**Two-piece dresses
  with own jacket**

Two or three from this group. Each garment good material, plain color, picking up fashion trend, starkly simple, crease-resistant, comfortable, and wearable from dawn to dusk.

Coats

*One all-purpose coat that would go with all the above and one double-duty coat.
Plain restrained colors, starkly simple.*

------

2 Basic accessories

**Scarves   Gloves   Shoes
Handbags**

*Black, white, or off-white, pale beige—these can generally be mixed in wear.
Go for* QUALITY *rather than quantity.*

------

3 Basic costume jewelry

**Necklaces   Bracelets
Brooches   Earrings**

*Collect first matching sets in pearl, pure white beads, jet, then in gold, silver, rhinestone, and real gems.
As a general rule wear matching or related pieces.*

------

4 Casuals

**Blouses   Sweaters
Skirts**

A small collection of these, interchangeable, and related in color to basic garments.

You have never finished your study of dress. There is always more to learn, new trends to follow, new fields to conquer (Paris, Rome, Florence, Dublin, London, when you've absorbed the home front). The subject becomes more and more fascinating and more rewarding as you grow older.

7 grooming

freshness, care of the body, clothes, and possessions

Freshness

Those advertisements... *her best friend wouldn't tell her...,...someone isn't using...* could refer to you and me and all of us. We are all perspiring over our whole body all the time, and we would not be healthy if we weren't. For the most part the perspiration is absorbed imperceptibly by clothes and the air, but underarm dampness must not be allowed for a second. Here is a list of musts:

1 Must keep dry.

2 Must keep clear of hair under arms and on legs.

3 Must use anti-perspirant deodorant.

4 Must follow implicitly the directions on the bottle—otherwise the product may not be able to do its work efficiently.

5 Must not get hot and risk perspiration during the time the product is drying off, as, again, the product may not be able to do its work efficiently.

6 Might have to change the brand she is using from time to time, because the body may develop a resistance to one particular brand after a while.

perfume

Although perfume is not a must for the well turned out young woman, I think we all feel that it provides that final extravagant touch that makes all the difference. If you decide to wear it, regard it rather as a lovely accessory to be used according to the time of the day and the occasion.

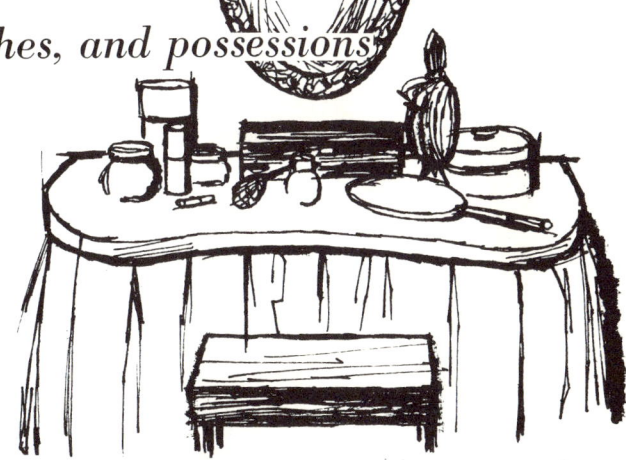

Ideally, the foundation of your fragrance should be laid during morning grooming by the use of matching perfumed soap, bath salts, toilet water, etc. This will give you an indefinable aura of freshness and fragrance throughout the day *and is enough* for a normal everyday environment. Just as the cocktail dress, however lovely, is out of place at 9 A.M. at the office, so is a strongly noticeable perfume. Away from your studies or your job, then you can allow yourself the sheer pleasure of adding matching scent—using sufficient to increase your perfume noticeably but not so much that you are drowned in it, which is considered very bad taste indeed. Incidentally, another good reason for being restrained is that the perfume you like may not be liked by others. It is wise to make sure in a tactful way that a person whose attachment you value *does* like the perfume you use.

Your personal choice of perfume will take time, and, let us face it, money—because good perfumes are made by experts from rare substances sought in the far-flung places of the earth, and they are therefore expensive. Do not hurry when selecting your first perfume. Preferably go to a counter where there is an expert to guide you. Learn to distinguish first between the light flower scents and the heavy exotic ones. Try to decide from which group you wish to select. Even then it may take you a year or so living with first one and then another until you find the one that satisfies you. Once this is achieved, then use this one only (until perhaps a few years later you feel the desire for a change) because there is something quite enchanting about being associated with a particular perfume.

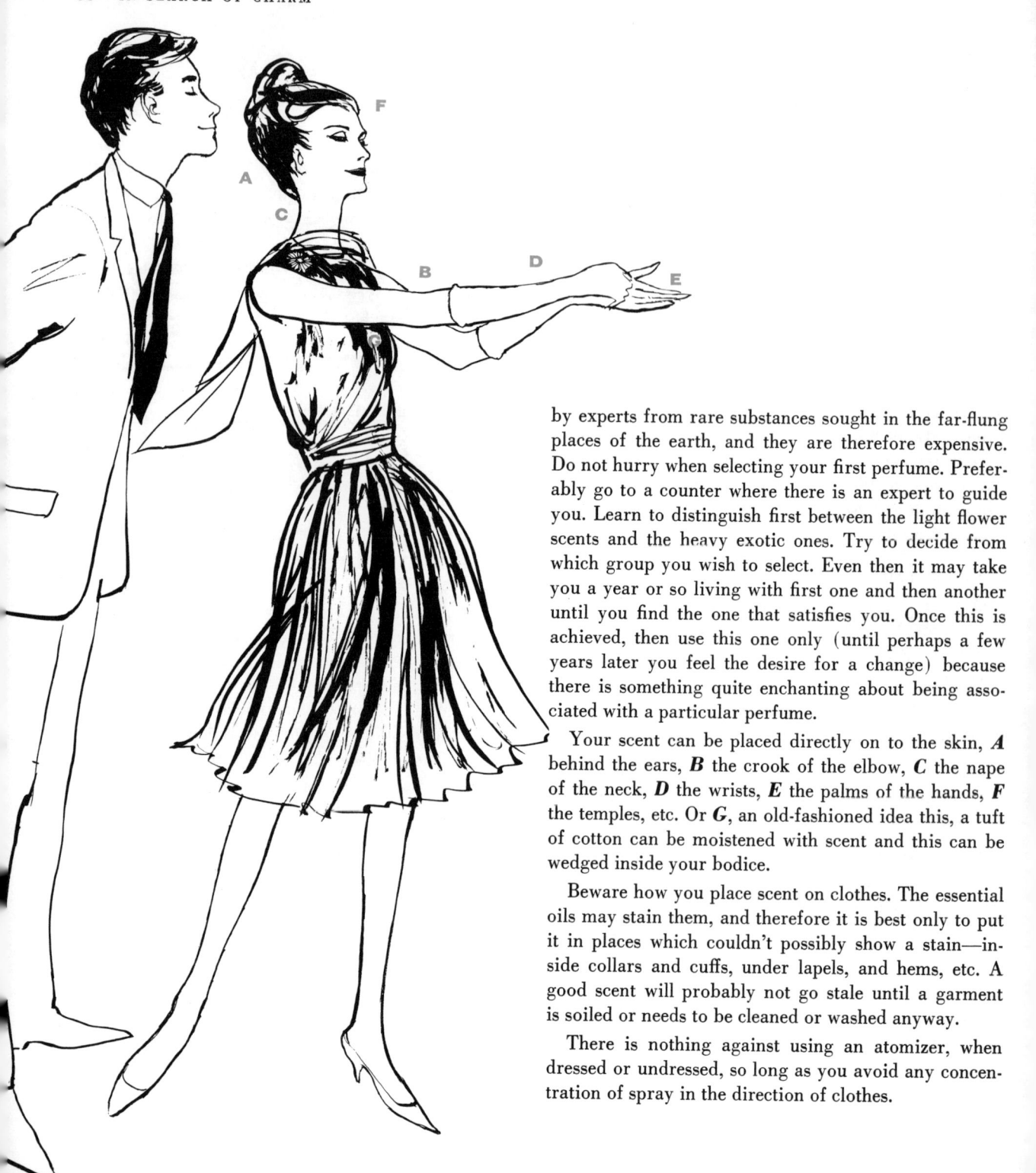

Your scent can be placed directly on to the skin, *A* behind the ears, *B* the crook of the elbow, *C* the nape of the neck, *D* the wrists, *E* the palms of the hands, *F* the temples, etc. Or *G*, an old-fashioned idea this, a tuft of cotton can be moistened with scent and this can be wedged inside your bodice.

Beware how you place scent on clothes. The essential oils may stain them, and therefore it is best only to put it in places which couldn't possibly show a stain—inside collars and cuffs, under lapels, and hems, etc. A good scent will probably not go stale until a garment is soiled or needs to be cleaned or washed anyway.

There is nothing against using an atomizer, when dressed or undressed, so long as you avoid any concentration of spray in the direction of clothes.

Body

Do you wake up dopey? Do you just give yourself a lick and a promise, gulp a cup of coffee, and creep out of the house half asleep? If so, here is the routine to combat all that.

in bed

Once you've opened your eyes, resist the temptation to close them again. Instead, fling arms above your head and stretch upwards through the body at least five times, finishing with each of the five fingers in turn. Then stretch downwards through the body to the toes in the same way. When you've counted out the last stretch, then without pausing to brood or think, turn back the bed clothes and get out of bed. Go through the stretching process all over again. All this takes about one-tenth of the time it has taken you to read about it.

and now to your bath

To be refreshing, this should be swift and vigorous and all completed in about five minutes. If you linger, you may become too relaxed. Scrub yourself vigorously all over (except for the complexion, which is dealt with quite separately) with a good mild soap and either a sponge or an old-fashioned bristle nailbrush. A nylon nailbrush is just a little too tough. Slide the body under the water for a few seconds—just long enough to rinse off the soap. In fact it's a good idea to start letting the water out before you slide under, and so remove the temptation to linger. Stand up in the bath and, while the water is still draining out of it, have either a cold shower or a cold sponge-down. The more shivery you tend to be and the colder the weather, *the more necessary* is the cold finish. The cold water is, of course, to close the pores. You must have experienced many times the warm body glow that follows a plunge into the swimming pool or the sea. Tell yourself not to be a baby about the cold water. Get on with it—it only takes five seconds.

After the cold rinse, remove surplus water quickly with a hand towel and only now climb out of the bath. Now follows a vigorous rubbing with a really rough towel until the body is pink with the friction—by which time it feels invigorated, glowing with warmth and health—and the skin is benefited too. By gripping the towel at each end, you can execute all kinds of to-and-fro horizontal and diagonal movements, plus much back bending when attacking the legs—all of which is excellent exercise in itself. By the time you put on clothes, you will feel wide awake and ready for anything. *And all this is in the normal* everyday course of getting up. I can assure you that once you have tried this routine, you will always want to start your day this way.

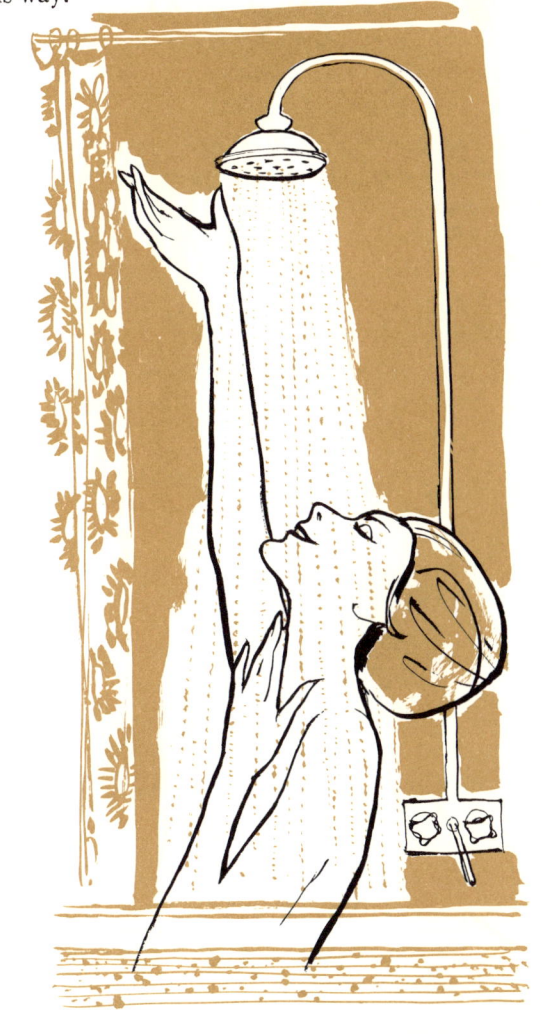

10 points about feet

Do you know?

1 That the state of your feet is reflected in the state of your health.

2 That tight, ill-fitting, uncomfortable shoes or neglected feet can actually make you feel irritable and bad-tempered.

3 That your feet can become half a size larger as the day wears on, particularly if you are standing a lot or if it is hot, and that therefore it's a good plan to change into comfortable shoes at midday.

4 That for general wear it is best to compromise between fashion and appearance by wearing, for instance, a neat, plain shoe with medium, neat heel. Thus you are comfortable and fairly smart too. It is a good plan to wear very high heels only when this seems to be essential for an occasion, and to wear flat-heeled shoes for walking any distance.

5 That too tight or too short stockings can cause foot troubles in the same way as do ill-fitting shoes.

6 That your feet should be scrubbed with soap and water and rinsed in cold water every morning and every night, and in fact as often as convenient. This is particularly necessary in hot weather.

7 That after washing, it is a good plan to treat your feet to a few seconds' massage, rubbing in as convenient some hand cream, skin food, oil or suntan lotion.

8 That hard skin should never be cut but dealt with by pumice stone (or its equivalent).

9 That toenails should be kept straightish and not shaped to curve down at the sides. This is to help keep them strong and to prevent ingrowing toenails and splintering.

10 That it is refreshing to change shoes and stockings during the day, and also to give the feet an airing. Take every opportunity of going barefoot, especially, of course, on vacation.

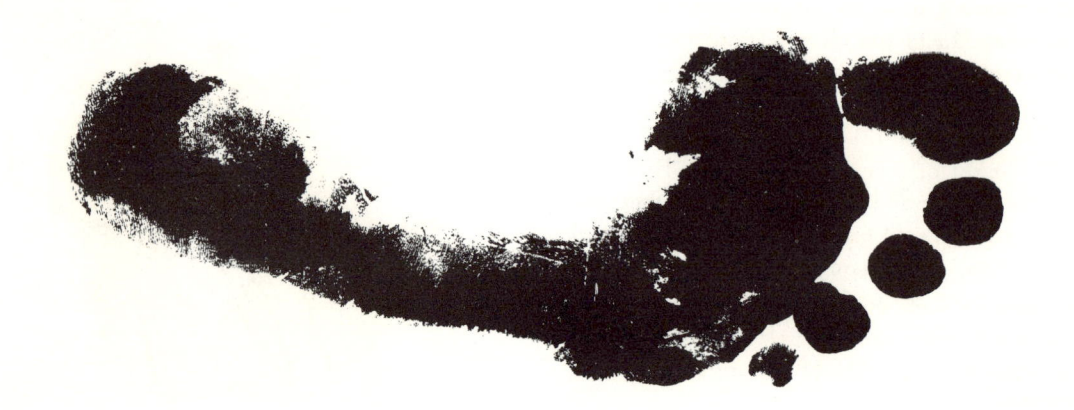

10 points about hands

Do you know?

1 That neglected hands and nails can undermine your confidence.

2 That some people will look at your hands and the way you use them as a guide to your character, health, and personality.

3 That it is best to have a regular weekly manicure *and* give your hands a little daily attention.

4 That hand creams and nail creams need to be under your nose in the bathroom and by the kitchen sink, otherwise you tend to forget to use them.

5 That it is best to leave weak or splitting nails alone as much as possible. Once they have been smoothed down by using an emery board on the flat, then put on a colorless wax base as a protection.

6 That simple, inexpensive mixtures such as colorless iodine with castor oil or lanolin with paraffin have been known to do wonders in restoring good strong nail growth. But remember that it's the new growth that becomes strengthened and therefore it is necessary to persevere with treatment patiently.

7 That it is best to avoid constant immersion of the hands in water—especially water containing any of the synthetic household soaps or detergents.

8 That you can buy thin rubber household gloves with a silkish lining. Therefore, if you have taken the trouble to massage in some oil or cream before putting on the gloves your hands can be having a beauty treatment while you are doing the household chores.

9 That if household gloves are really impossible for a job, then a protective cream is a must. This is particularly necessary for a girl doing an office job entailing the handling of typewriter ribbons, duplicating machines, etc.

10 That the expression "prevention is better than cure" is especially applicable in the case of hands—because a cure may take weeks—and that is too late for a date with the boy friend for tonight.

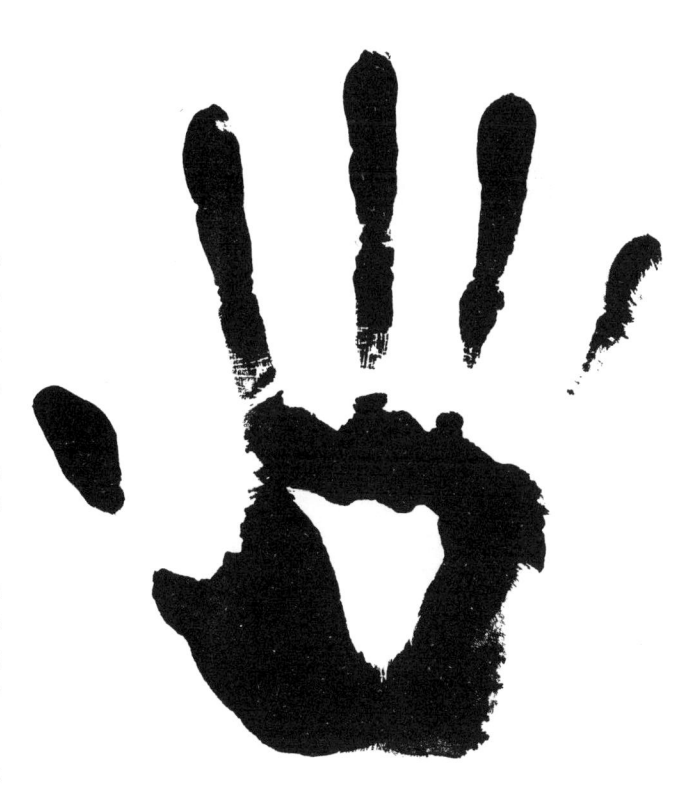

5 points about legs

Do you know?

1 That nothing looks more unsightly than a growth of dark hair showing through your sheer stockings.

2 That when you have to kneel to do certain exercises or to do household chores, then some pliant kneeling surface should be used. It is quite extraordinary how quickly knees can look roughened.

3 That in any case it is advisable to give your knees a little massage from time to time. You can always spare a little hand cream or skin food for this purpose.

4 That if your legs have to be on view for, say, a part in a play or in fancy dress costume, and yet you are bothered because they are looking patchy or pallid, they can steal the show if you use some stage leg make-up on them.

5 That in the summer you should try to get your legs brown first because they tend to take longer to brown than the rest of the body. They are, as it were, more acclimatized to sun, wind, and rain by being merely clad for most of the year in thin stockings.

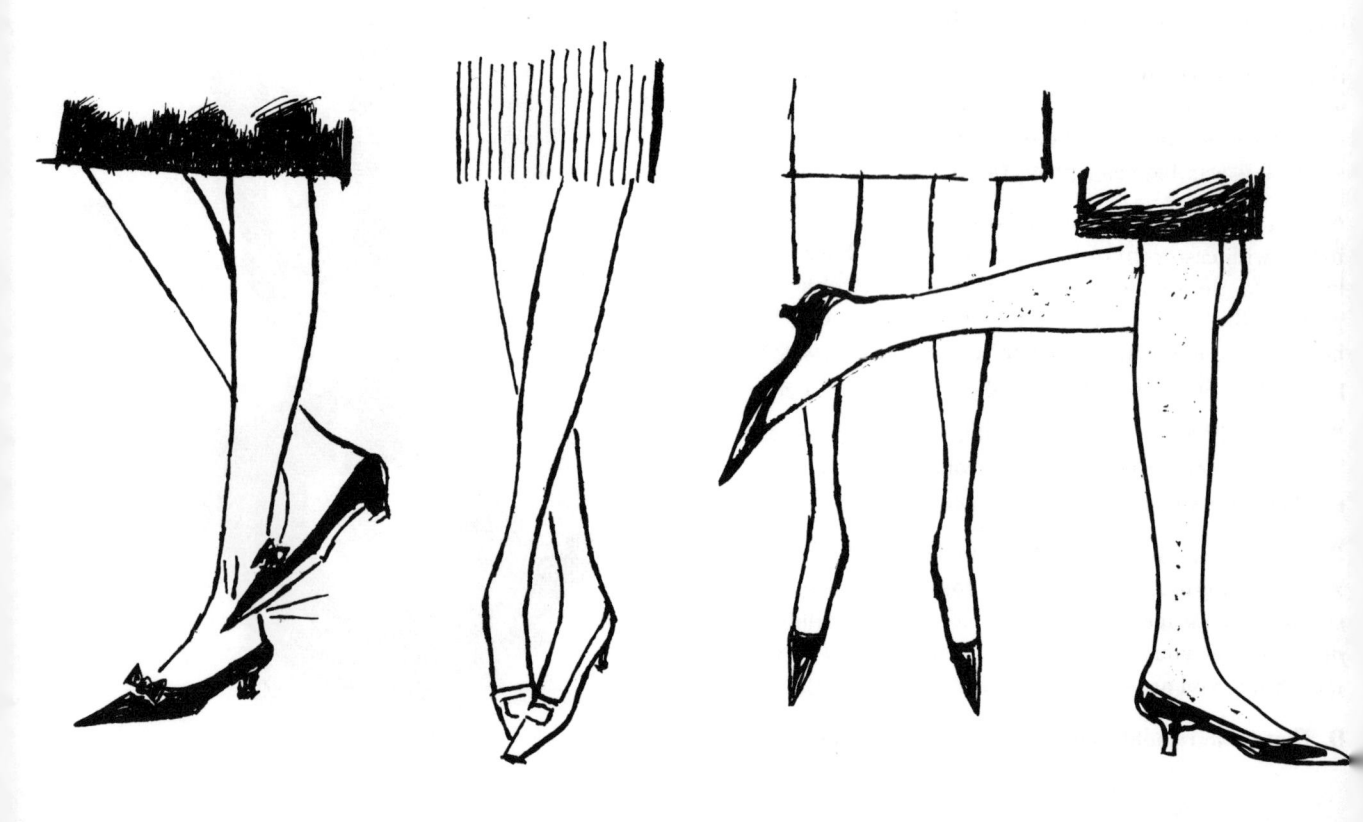

10 points about hair and scalp

Do you know?

1 That on getting up (and as part of your normal routine when starting to do your hair for the day), it is a good thing to bend over with the head hanging down and pull and pull at the roots until the whole scalp is tingling. This attracts circulation to the roots, as well as helping in that process of waking you up.

2 That you should then massage the scalp for a minute or so by *moving it*. Place the palms of the hands firmly on the scalp and let one palm hold on firmly while the other one pushes the scalp around. Keep switching over the functions of the palms and changing their position until you have worked over the whole of the scalp.

3 That it is best to brush the hair in long strokes from root to tip, and again, for the most part with the head bending over and well down. Brush, followed by hand, brush, hand, and so on.

4 That if you want to keep a reputation for shining hair, then shampoo it *the day before* you know it is likely to look its worst.

5 That if you're really no good at managing your own hair, then make up your mind to pay a regular visit to the hairdresser for shampooing and setting and *keeping in a good shape*. Shape is everything.

6 That you risk ruining your hair when you bleach without regard to what is happening to its texture.

7 That you also risk ruining your hair when you madly try out new products without first finding out whether they are suitable for *your* hair—or suitable after some special hair treatment.

8 That you risk ruining your hair, too, when you rush to dyes before having professional advice and a test for allergy.

9 That back-combing itself doesn't do your hair any harm, but any vicious form of combing out can.

10 That on vacation, your hair needs some sort of protection (a large kerchief or big shady hat or both together, which is an intriguing combination) against prolonged exposure to hot sunshine, which can act as a powerful bleaching and drying agent. Of course, the use of a conditioning cream will help to counteract this to some extent.

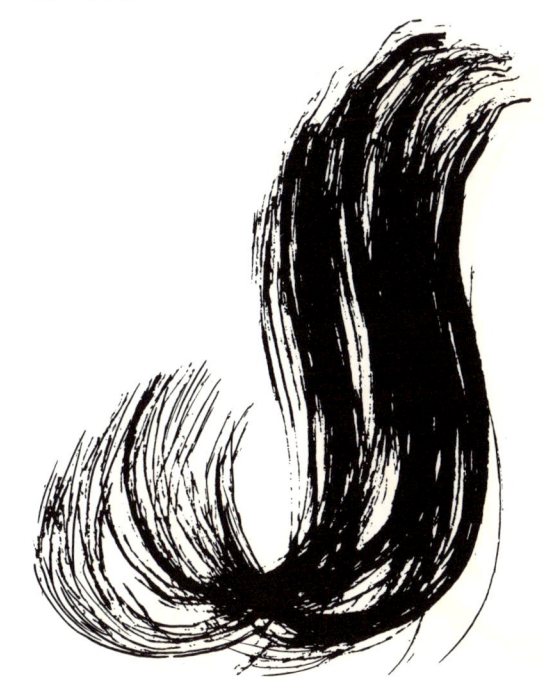

Hair styles

If you have lovely hair and an architecturally beautiful face and head, it probably doesn't matter what hair style you wear. This is the sort of beauty which movie stars must have. It is necessary for them to look equally beautiful in a period or modern style, when drowning or in the middle of a wildcat fight. Very few of us have this kind of beauty, and therefore the sooner we find out what we can and cannot do with our hair, the happier we will be.

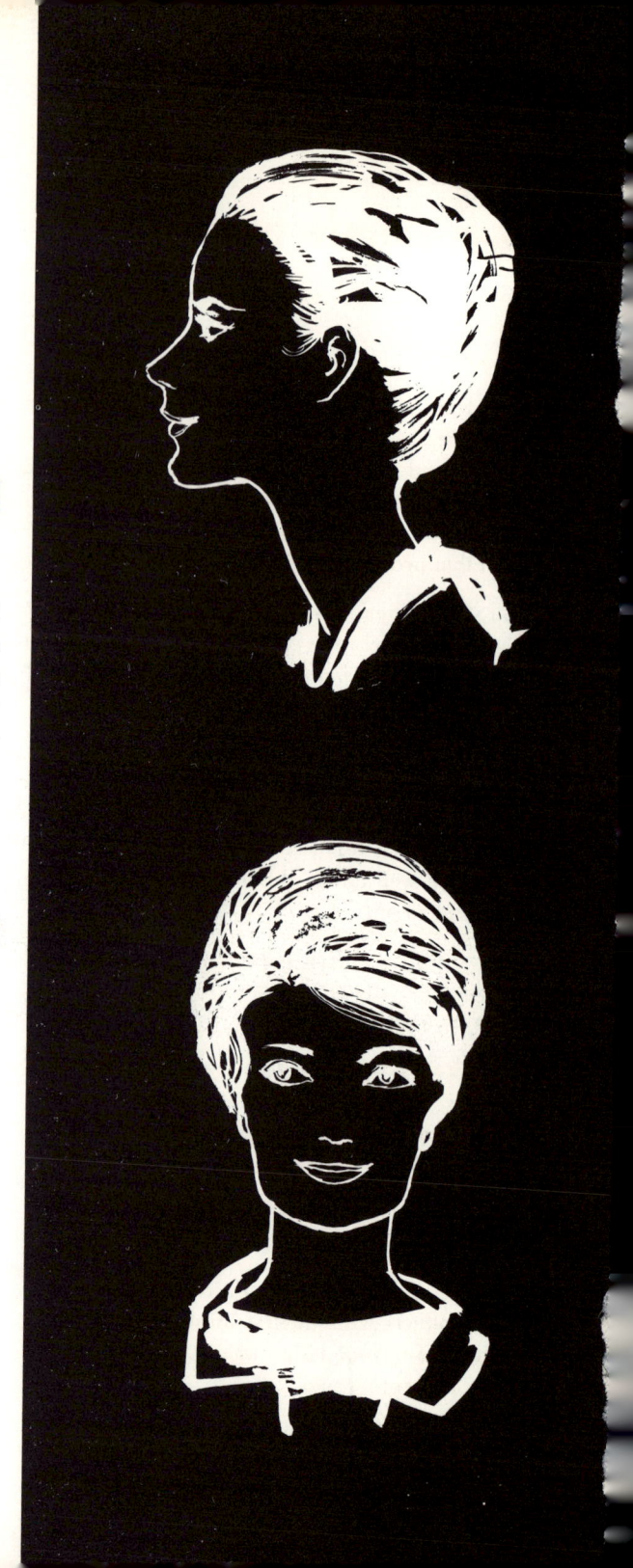

large head

With a LARGE HEAD, the fluffed-out or over-bouffant style that will make the head look even larger should be avoided. A smooth, head-hugging style will be most effective.

small head

A SMALL HEAD with a good head of hair is no problem. A small head with fine hair needs something to give a little bulk. Try a permanent wave and a bouffant style. A small head with long fine hair worn up can be given extra bulk by the use of foundations and switches.

broad jaw

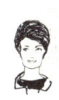

If you have a BROAD JAW, avoid hair width just at the line where the jaw is broad. A wave covering part of the jaw may help, but width at the temples and height on top of the head will best counteract and frame the breadth of jaw. The interest on top will create good balance.

high forehead

A HIGH FOREHEAD isn't something to conceal at all costs. Provided that the hairline is good, then an upswept, off-the-brow style can look fabulous. However, if the hairline is not good and if you tend to look bald with your hair swept back, then avoid this scraped-up look by concealing and flattering the high forehead either by a wispy, tendrilly, or curly fringe, or by setting all the top hair forward from the crown so that when brushed back it will respond to being eased forward to cover and soften the hairline.

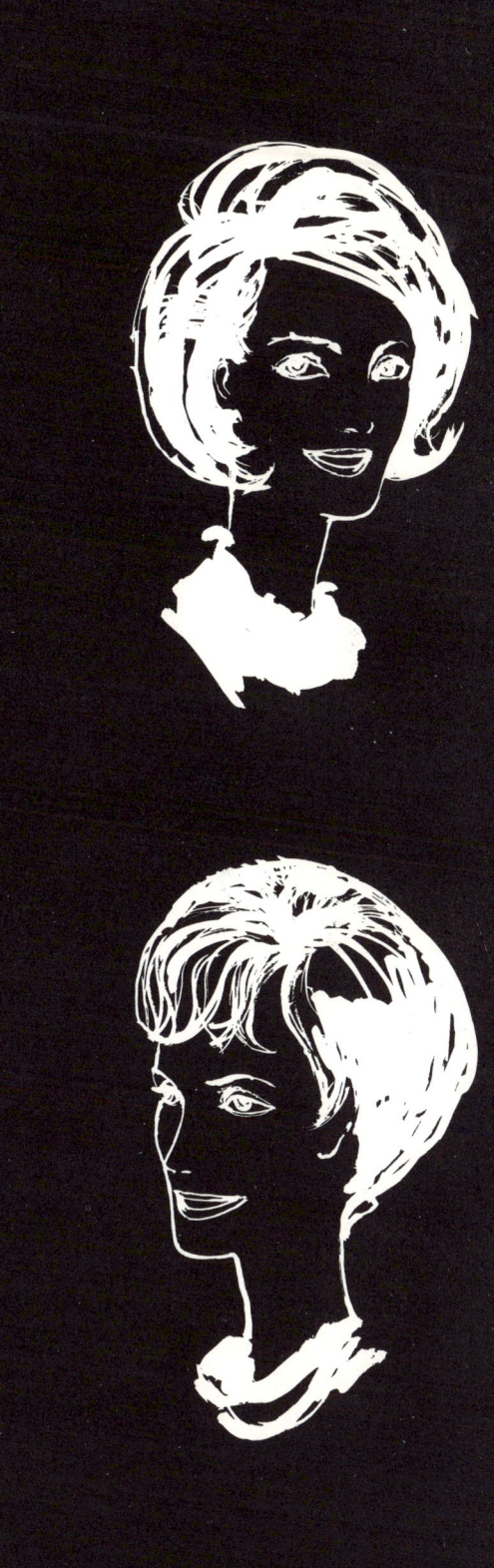

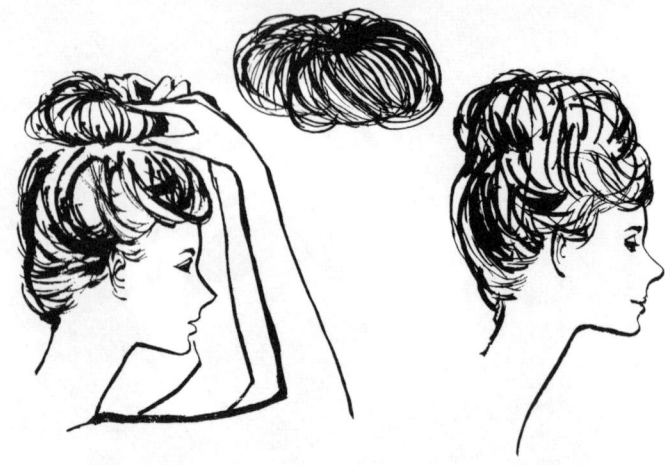

Having read thus far, you may be groaning because your problem is a mixture of several difficult features. Well, I know one model who has successfully, after quite a deal of experiment, solved her complex problem of small flat head, small face with broadish jaw, high forehead with poor hairline and fine hair. This is how she did it.

(*a*) She had a permanent wave to give the hair body and then just let it grow.

(*b*) As soon as it had lost its shape and had gained a little length, she *brushed* it all up towards the top of the head; then arranged the hair around the face in a beret style. She found this easing of the hair over the hairline did more for her face than did a fringe, which seemed to drown her small face.

(*c*) She then wound a largish matching nylon switch into a soft bun and pinned it on top of the head, spreading out fronds of the switch to catch any short ends of hair. This height and bulk on top did more than anything to counteract the effect of the small flat head and broad jaw.

(*d*) When the hair had enough length, she began experimenting by putting the switch (broken down into two parts by now) partly under her own hair, or in different positions and arrangements. Her ambition is that eventually she will be able to manage without a switch at all. All this may sound a little complicated, but this model now has a distinctive Suzie Wong, slightly old-world style all her own, which is elegant, and which she finds more manageable than any of the short styles she used to battle with. Moreover, the switch on top controls all that fine flying soft hair. If *you* have been yearning to put up your hair, but yet feel you haven't the looks for it, then this can be quite a formula for achieving a soft, becoming style.

Clothes and possessions

Would your wardrobe and drawers bear inspection, or are all your things tumbled and jumbled up inside? Is your room always a litter of shoes that need cleaning, stockings that need washing, and odd garments that have just been dumped here and there?

The counsel of perfection (as laid down in all the best beauty books) is a place for everything and tidy as you go. First of all, organize that place for everything. Spring clean every drawer, closet, shelf, and wardrobe. Next, collect all articles together, deciding broadly which can be folded into piles, which must be laid out in a drawer, and which must be hung up. Then economically allot the space you have available. When you have finally arranged all this, keeping *all* gloves together, *all* shoes together, *all* blouses together, *all* sweaters neatly folded together in one pile, etc., you will not only know where everything is, but it will give you much pleasure just to survey the result of your trouble.

WHAT ABOUT YOUR HANDBAG? Is it full of old tickets, dog-eared envelopes, uncared-for combs, and cosmetics, not to mention hair clips, money, and keys all mixed up together?

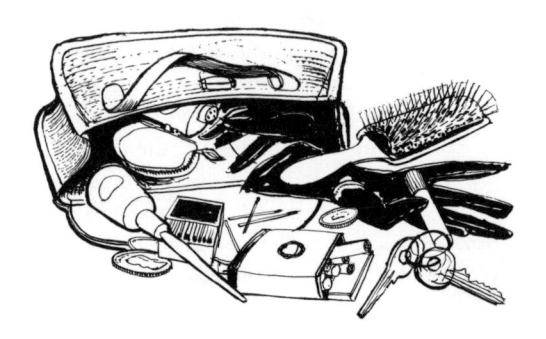

At the end of the day, turn out, dust, and put away your bag (in a neat row on a shelf with the others, of course). Then, on a small tray specially reserved for this purpose in one corner of a shelf or drawer, place the hard-core of your handbag requirements, making sure that they are put there in immaculate condition. There they are the following morning ready to be gathered up and placed in the handbag for the day.

As soon as you take off your shoes, put in shoe-trees, and either set them ready for cleaning, or clean them immediately and then put them away. Examine shoes daily for repair needs. Heels should be repaired long before they have that down-at-the-heel look.

Coats, suits, dresses should be brushed, and have any marks removed from them when you take them off. Then hang them up in such a way that they fall correctly. Avoid coat-hangers which push out the material.

Presumably most of your undies are nylon. So why not swish them straight away through slightly soapy water, rinse them, and hang them up to drip-dry overnight!

Toilet articles(brushes, combs, cosmetics, nailbrush, washcloth, etc.) should be kept immaculate as you go along.

If you follow all these ideas, you should have no accumulation of putting away, washing, brushing, and stain or mark removing, and your routine of getting dressed in the morning becomes a real joy as you just collect all your requirements.

Despite all this, it is still necessary to give yourself a final inspection before setting out:

Loose hairs?
Dandruff?
Dust or lint?
Buttons secure and properly fastened?
Shoulder straps properly tethered by lingerie loops or clips?
Stocking seams straight?
Shoes immaculate?

This chapter seems to spell much hard work, but remember the old French maxim that to be beautiful, you have to suffer. However, you will find that the hard work will be considerably eased if you are continuously streamlining your activities and routines. In course of time you will find that this disciplined organization of yourself, of your wardrobe, and of your possessions will automatically go into action, and with what pride and joy you will do it all when you visit friends, when you travel, and above all when you get married.

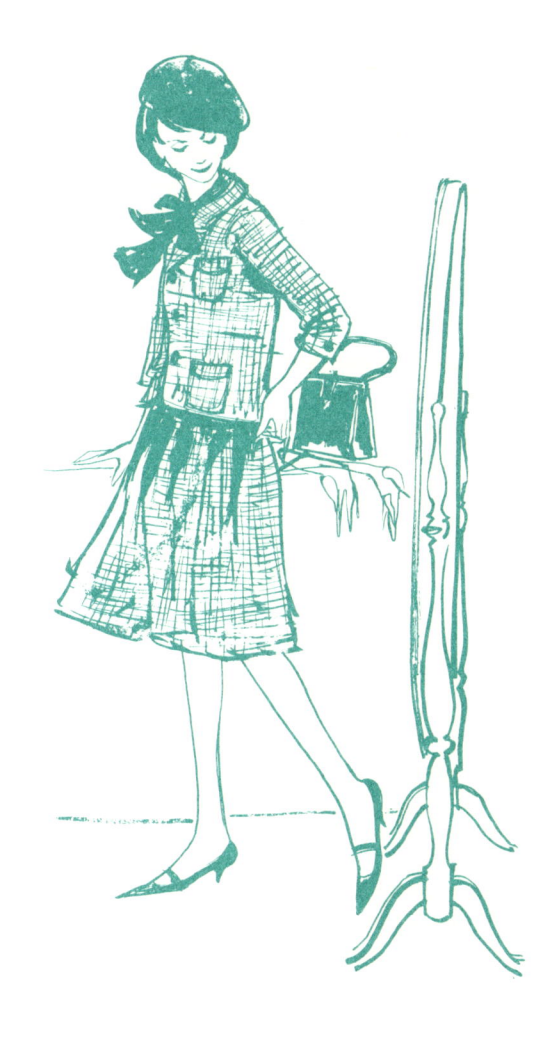

8 personality

There may come a moment in your life, if in fact it hasn't come already, when you're suddenly aware of personality in someone. For myself I can certainly pinpoint the moment and the person, and from then on I yearned to have some special quality myself. And yet if you *have* personality, you will hardly be aware of it because it is so much part and parcel of being yourself. It will be, rather like beauty, in the eye of the beholder.

The more you think about it, the more you realize that personality defies analysis. A child, a bird, a dog can have it. We speak of a pale personality, a vivid personality, and after all, if you could think of the devil as a person, he too would certainly have personality.

Amid this diversity, and in the context of this book, let us agree that your existing personality will grow and be enriched as you *strive* along your own lines. All I can do is offer guidance.

If you have been taking your family and closest friends for granted, try observing them a little more closely. Perhaps they need a little more of your time and help.

Have you been keeping pace with what is happening in your county, your town or city, your country, the world? You can't follow closely everything that is going on, but you can keep a general picture in your mind by reading the headlines and important articles in your newspapers, and listening to or looking at radio and television news reports.

Once you have tuned yourself in to current events, you can usually tune in to any conversation or discussion anywhere. Start by listening and then asking a few modest questions. As and when you can, visit the movies, theater, concerts, the ballet, choosing those programs which have aroused controversy among the critics as well as those which provide easy entertainment.

Traveling abroad widens your horizons, and so does reading. Biographies can be particularly rewarding, as you learn of the trials and tribulations of personalities of the past. Until you have confidence in your powers of conversation, I suggest you could quite deliberately prepare ahead subjects for introducing into conversation before evenings out or parties. Set out to meet new people with the idea that they may be feeling *more* shy, *more* reserved, than you yourself and that it is *your job* to draw out out people and make them feel they are interesting. In tackling the very reserved looking people you may have to try several of your subjects ("Did you see on television this ... or that?," "Have you been away yet?," "Have you read ... ?" etc.), but once you get some response, then fan the flame by being ready with the sort of questions that start with the words who, what, why, when, where. Be ashamed to be the one whom others have to draw out. During the course of a party, let it be a matter of pride with you that you talk to almost everyone there. A party is not the place in which to get bogged down in a corner for hours and hours.

Whatever your hobbies and leisure activities, join a group or club associated with them. Tennis clubs, dramatic societies, musical societies, literary groups, and so on, all offer their members scope for their activities as well as providing a certain amount of social life. But join with the idea of being one of the most active members, even if you do take on a little more than you think you can manage, and even if you do take on responsibility for speaking up at some meeting, or taking part in some play, when you have never done these things before. It may well be that at the time of having to do either of these things, your knees will knock together. Take no notice of this; in time they will not knock so much, if at all. And when you reach that stage, what more proof will you need that you have developed?

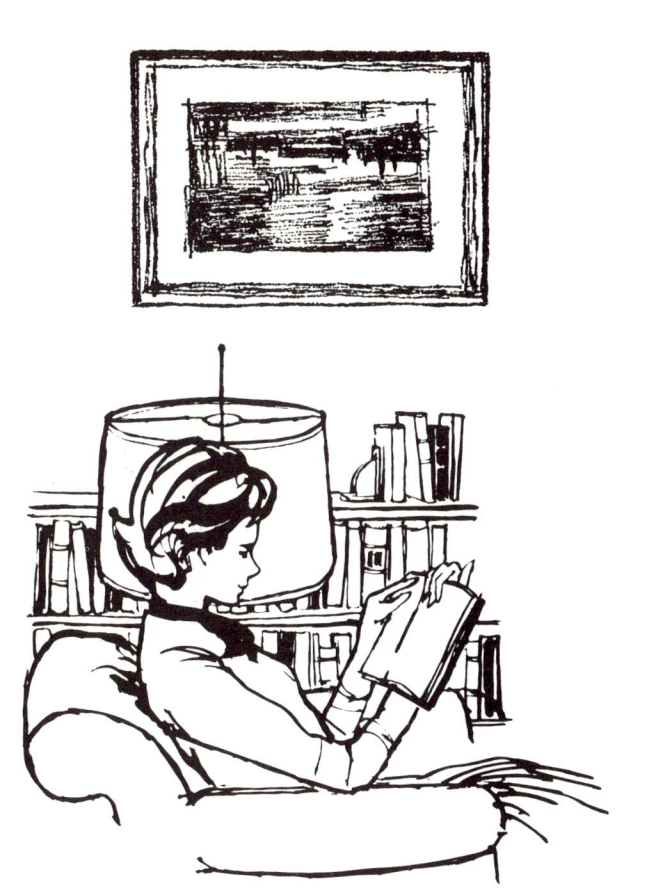

Don't let your brain stagnate: the more you use it, the more you *can* use it and, therefore, I suggest that you should be studying at least one subject all the time. The practical course of action is to enroll in a course which will help you in your career, or in your hobbies, or in a subject about which you know you are embarrassingly ignorant. Learning a language never fails to help you later on, either for business or for vacations (or both). As time goes on, as I discovered for myself, your most unlikely studies of today can make all the difference to your qualifications for a job tomorrow. Inexpensive evening courses are available everywhere, and information about these is to be had for the asking at public libraries or schools. The courses of the one I happen to have in front of me at this moment (I teach "Poise, Dress and Personality" for this one) ranges through cooking, dressmaking, flower arranging, drama, first aid, languages, folk dancing, Spanish dancing, public speaking, travel, physical training, music, ballroom dancing, ballet, photography, and so on; it is really incredible how much is offered.

Reading books (and I mean *books* rather than magazines) can bring confidence through knowledge, as well as enjoyment. Whatever your interest, there is bound to be a book on the subject. You can read in the newspapers descriptions and reviews of the books which everyone is talking about. Borrow them from your library so that you can form your own opinion.

Finally, build up your own *personal* library in your home. Books give a room that lived-in look and are attractive decorations in themselves too. And remember that these days the whole range of the world's literature and knowledge is available in paperback books, which cost no more, and often less, than the price of a good movie.

Self-reliance and dependability

Equip yourself with street maps, railroad and bus maps and timetables, and learn to look things up for yourself.

Find out the north, south, east, and west of your house, your locality, your town or city, and of every new place to which you go. (This is the clue to getting yourself around in the right direction. It will be equally helpful in getting around Paris, Rome, and London, when you are fortunate enough to be able to go to these far-flung cities.)

Wherever you are, whatever you are doing, always have paper and pencil ready. Any minute it may be vital to write something down (such as an address, a telephone number, the name of a piece of music to which you are listening, or the title of a book). It goes without saying that this is necessary when answering a telephone, whether you are at home, in business, or in a public phone booth.

You are a nuisance to yourself and everyone around, too, if you are forever having to conduct a search for your keys, your money, and change. Try keeping these things together in one small purse inside your main handbag.

Keep, too, in this purse *one small piece of notepaper* (neatly folded to fit in). Label one side Home and the other side Away. Put down *as they occur to you* on their appropriate side, in neatly headed lists, all the things you may forget to do. Thus every time you have to get out money or keys, there is a reminder to attend to all those small matters which must be done if life is to run smoothly and with peace of mind. You will be surprised how the items on the lists do get attended to—and with what joy every few days you will be transferring the leftovers to a fresh sheet. This little system should cut out the habit which some of you may have of continually asking others to remind you about this and that. This is not exactly being self-reliant and it can be very irritating.

First things first

As you develop and your interests widen, life can become very full, and there are bound to come times when you seem to be surrounded by six or seven matters all claiming your immediate attention. This need never get you down if you have trained yourself to put first things first. Thus the important things get done, and if time runs out, it is only the less important things which get left. This is certainly the golden rule in any well-conducted office, where there are usually many urgent tasks taking daily precedence and then quite a number of tasks to be caught up with when a busy period is over.

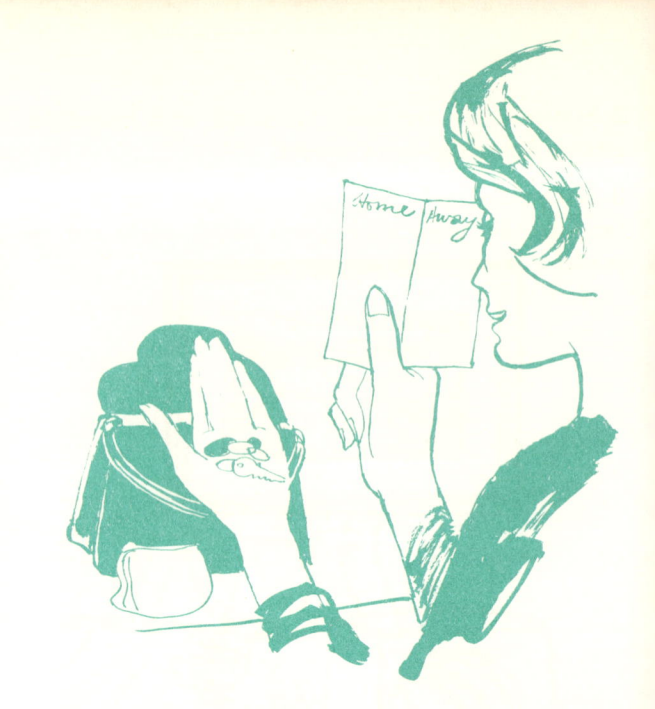

Double precautions

The application of the idea means different things to different people. To me it means such things as the following:

1 Taking spare accessories (such as stockings, gloves, costume jewelry) on important occasions. This is particularly necessary in my case. I would be embarrassed to appear on a platform to talk about grooming and dress if I had a run in my stocking, a soiled glove, or broken jewelry, and any of these mishaps could occur during the course of a journey. For similar reasons, I hardly ever leave home in the summer without my nylon raincoat (with matching headwear) which folds practically into a big envelope, and a collapsible umbrella. Since I always carry spare shoes and it is usually necessary for me to have cosmetics and business papers with me, I solve the problem by carrying everything in one large, plain, elegant bag that is right with my outfit.

2 Systematically replacing personal and household articles *before* they have run out.

3 Having not only the regulation spare tire for the car, but also other vital spares which might not be available in out-of-the-way places.

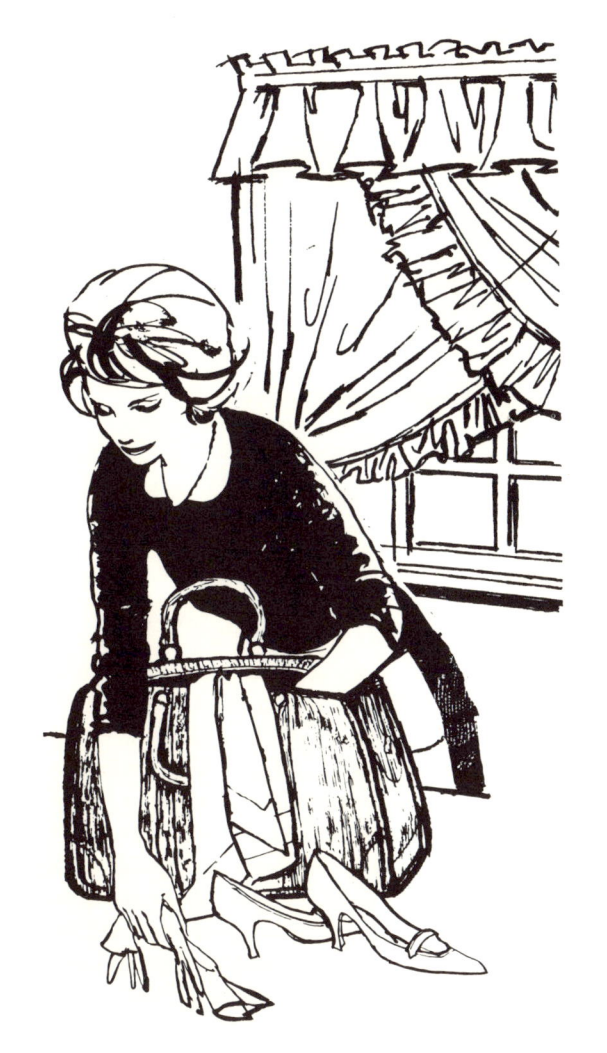

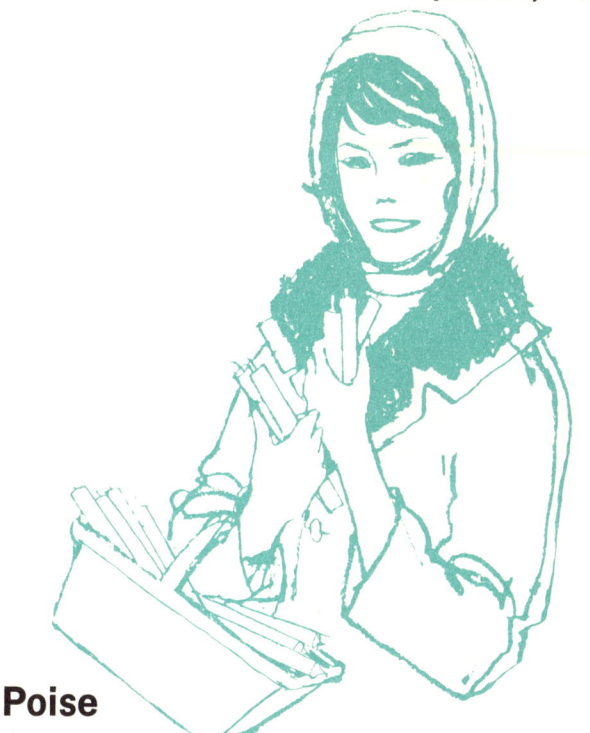

Poise

I am hoping that by now you will have discovered for yourself the calming effect on mind and body of an orderly, well-conducted, knowing-what-you-are-doing way of living. However, there is still the possibility of unexpected worries, special anxieties, and difficult decisions. If these are not to upset your equilibrium and ruin your sleep (and therefore your looks), you do need to have some very definite way of dealing with them.

Try spending just two minutes every night of your life just before dropping off to sleep quietly stating to yourself in *clear, plain language* just what are the matters on your mind—problem number one, problem number two, and so on, placing them mentally in strict order of importance. Then snuggle down to your sleep with the one thought that you will sleep on your problems and that you will wake up the following morning a little nearer to solving them. This is a technique that you will probably develop in your own way, and that you will find is not far removed from what is understood by meditation or prayer.

9 voice and laughter

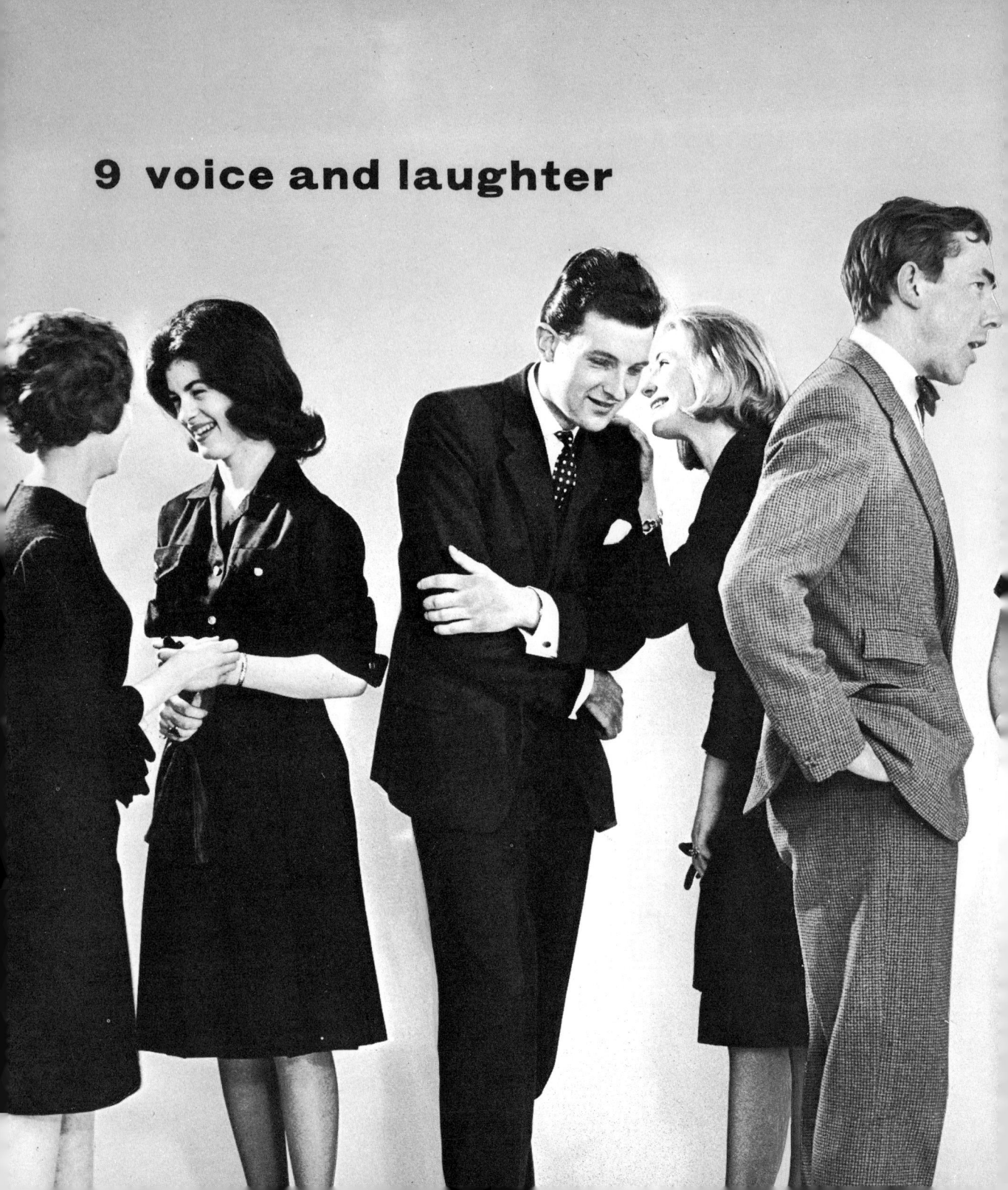

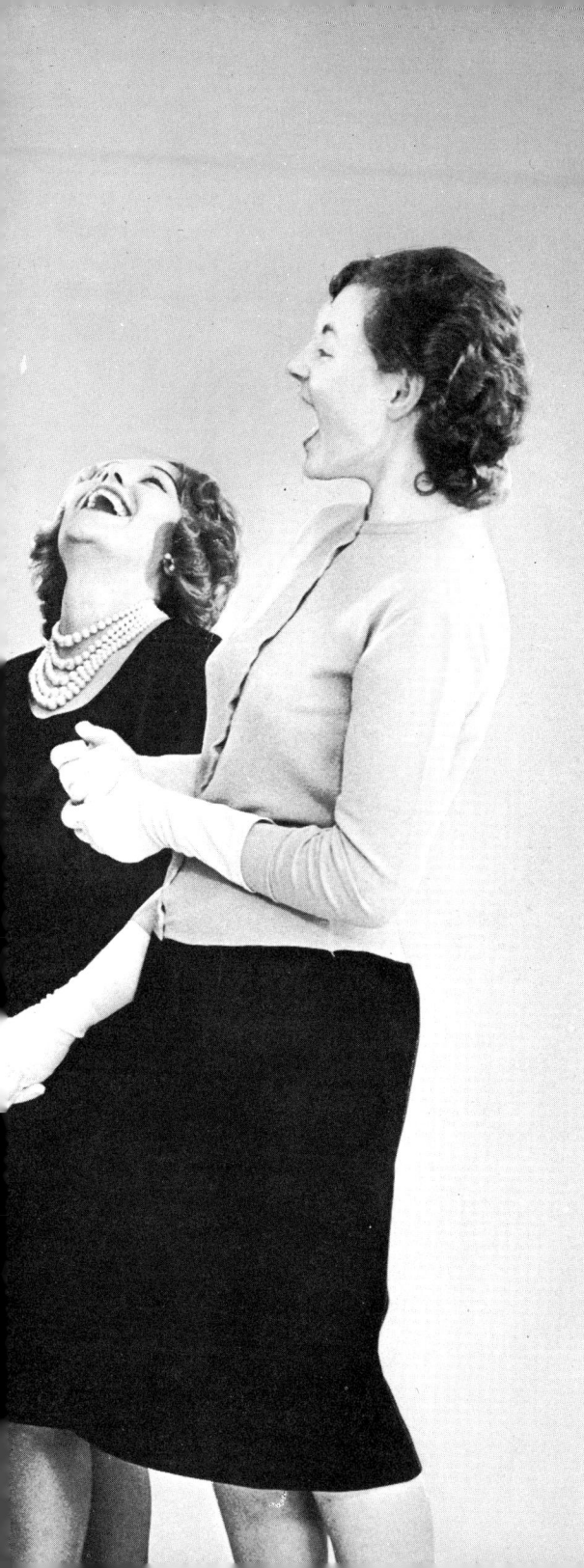

giggling

This is quite embarrassing both to yourself and to others. In fact, some people will consider it discourteous. You know from experience that the more you give in to it, the more you seem to be possessed by it. If you can, go away by yourself to recover your equilibrium. Certainly go away from the person with whom you are sharing giggles.

whispering

This looks bad from any point of view. You risk being thought rude, bored, or even malicious. The worst version is whispering behind the hand.

talking too much

This is always considered to be a very feminine fault, although between you, me, and the gatepost, men are just as guilty. It is wise to ask yourself if what you are saying:

(a) is really worth while
(b) could possibly be of interest to others
(c) could be boring others
(d) could be expressed more concisely or clearly?

talking too loudly

This can be unfeminine, self-centered, and inconsiderate.

using slang and swear words

This is also unfeminine and most unattractive. Moreover, some people will consider it all a deliberate act.

infuriating to live with

A raucous voice
A deadly, monotonous voice
A high-pitched voice
A mumbling voice
Indirect replies to questions
Long-winded replies to questions—with the answer at the remote end.

Sudden noisy shouts
Sudden noisy laughter
Talking to people from another room
Talking to people while you are walking away.

Speaking tips

Make an effort to send the voice in the direction of the person, or people, to whom you are speaking. In conversation, allow other people to finish what they are saying before you speak. In general try to respond to what they are saying, don't just ignore completely their subject and jump in with what you have been impatiently saving up to say.

Be sure you gain attention before, or as, you speak. For instance, don't rush into a room bursting out with six or seven sentences quite regardless of whether the person to whom you are addressing your remarks is concentrating on something else (such as writing a letter or speaking on the telephone). All that happens is that the person has to ask you to start all over again.

Voice confidence

This will increase if you will read aloud regularly. Start in the privacy of your bedroom. Stand up and read out one paragraph from a book or newspaper. If you read it badly, then keep on reading it (ten times if necessary) until you have finally read it in fairly good style. Do this every day for a while until you feel more confident of your voice. Then ask a friend if she will play audience for you. The more self-conscious you feel about this, the more you need to do it. (You will probably discover, as with many things, that the perfection you reach in the privacy of your room is difficult to maintain before others.)

In addition, listen attentively to good speakers on radio and television programs. Notice the well-formed vowels, the crisp consonants, and the phrasing.

However, if you don't speak well, if your voice is unattractive, or if you have no confidence in the sound of your own voice, then nothing will take the place of going to a trained teacher or enrolling in a speech-training course, and making up your mind that it will be necessary to attend regularly until you have improved.

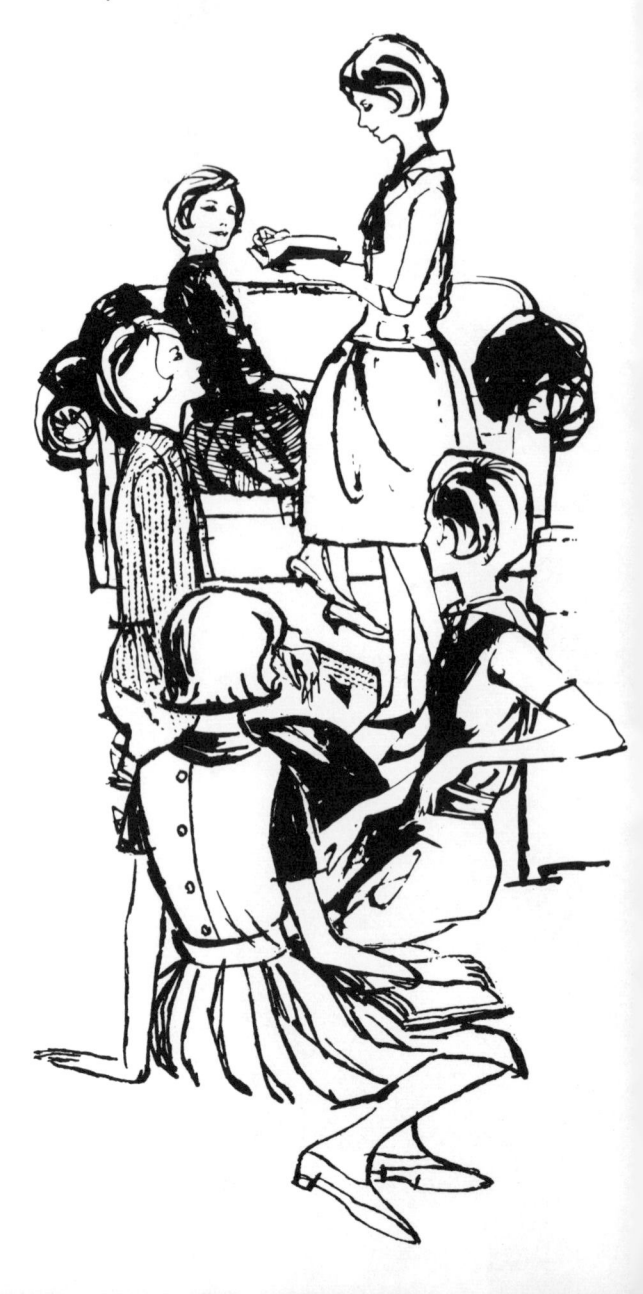

10 etiquette and behavior

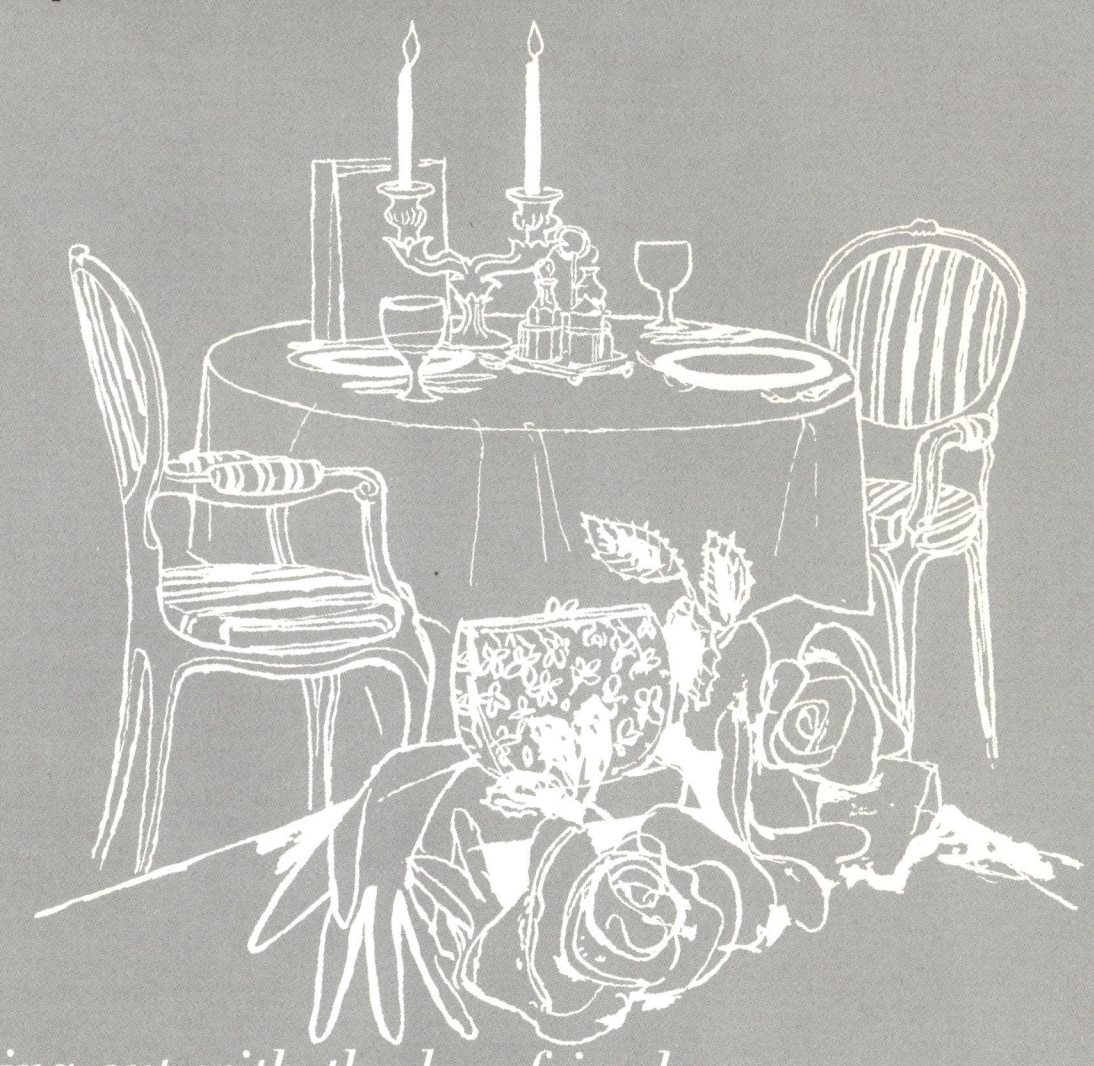

an evening out with the boy friend
INCLUDING A MEAL AT A RESTAURANT

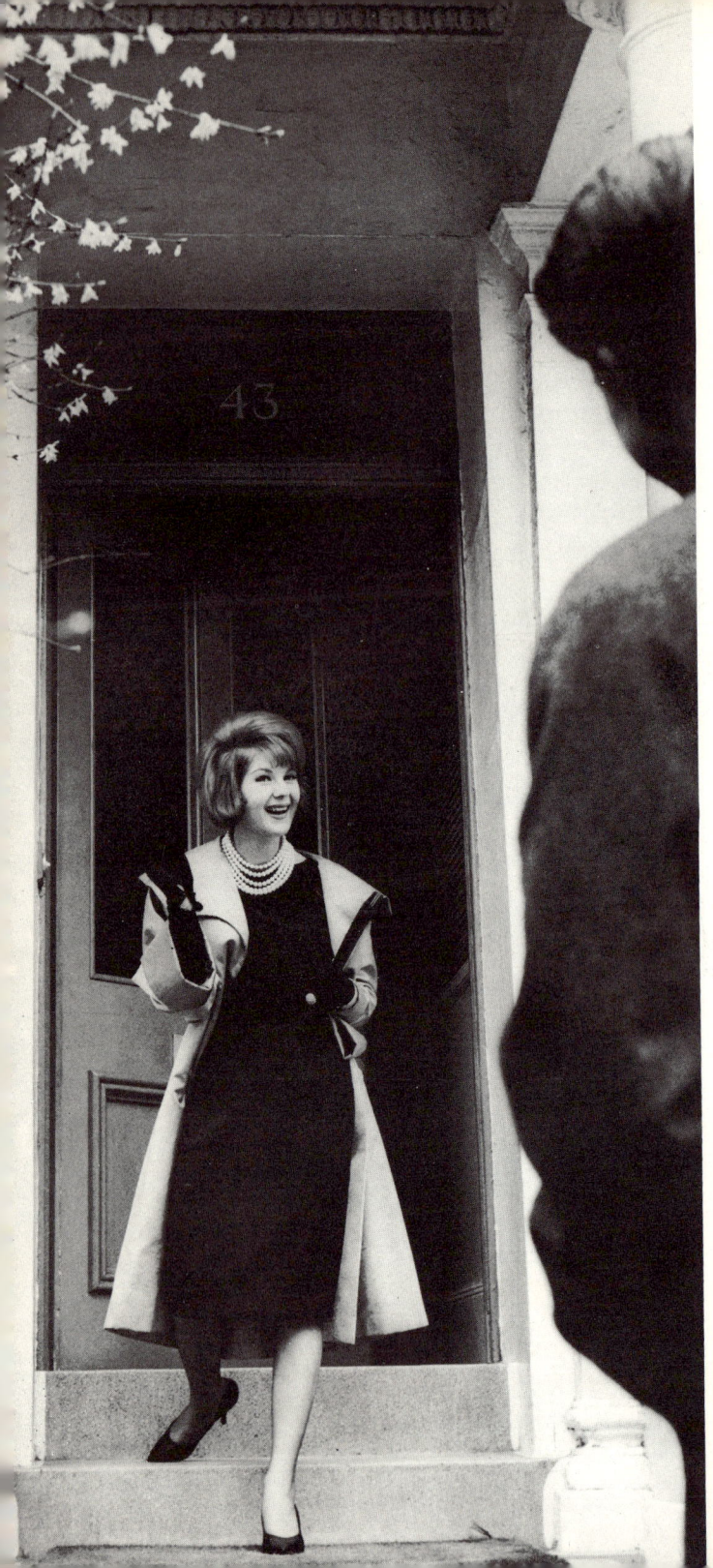

Common sense, consideration for others, and a certain fastidiousness are reliable guides to behavior anywhere. Additionally, down the years social custom has built up a multitude of musts and must-nots. Since many reliable volumes have been written on this subject, ranging from guidance on etiquette at christenings right through life's social occasions to guidance on etiquette at funerals, in this chapter I shall just try to give you some very general guidance for everyday happenings.

what to wear

Choose the little black number (or its equivalent) which will go anywhere (barring a full evening-dress occasion). If you have to wear it during the day, then you could have some glamorous accessories into which to change for the evening.

what to carry

Just a small, neat handbag holding minimum requirements of makeup, money, etc., is all you need. A large handbag full of cosmetics, personal papers, letters, a lot of cash, etc., will not only look out of place but you will hardly dare to put it down for a minute, even if there is an opportunity for dancing. Don't be laden down with parcels. Apart from the fact that these will ruin your appearance (you should of course present a picture of uncluttered, serene radiance), your escort may take one look at you and inwardly groan, knowing it will be his job to do all the carrying.

where to meet

Ideally, your escort should call for you at home. As this is often impracticable these days, then arrange to meet at your place of work, a theater, restaurant, or hotel. Avoid meeting in the street. Arrive one or two minutes late (certainly not more than five minutes late) because ideally your escort should be there *waiting for you*, and he may well be concerned if he finds that *you* are waiting for *him*. If he is late, assume it was unavoidable.

etiquette and behavior 77

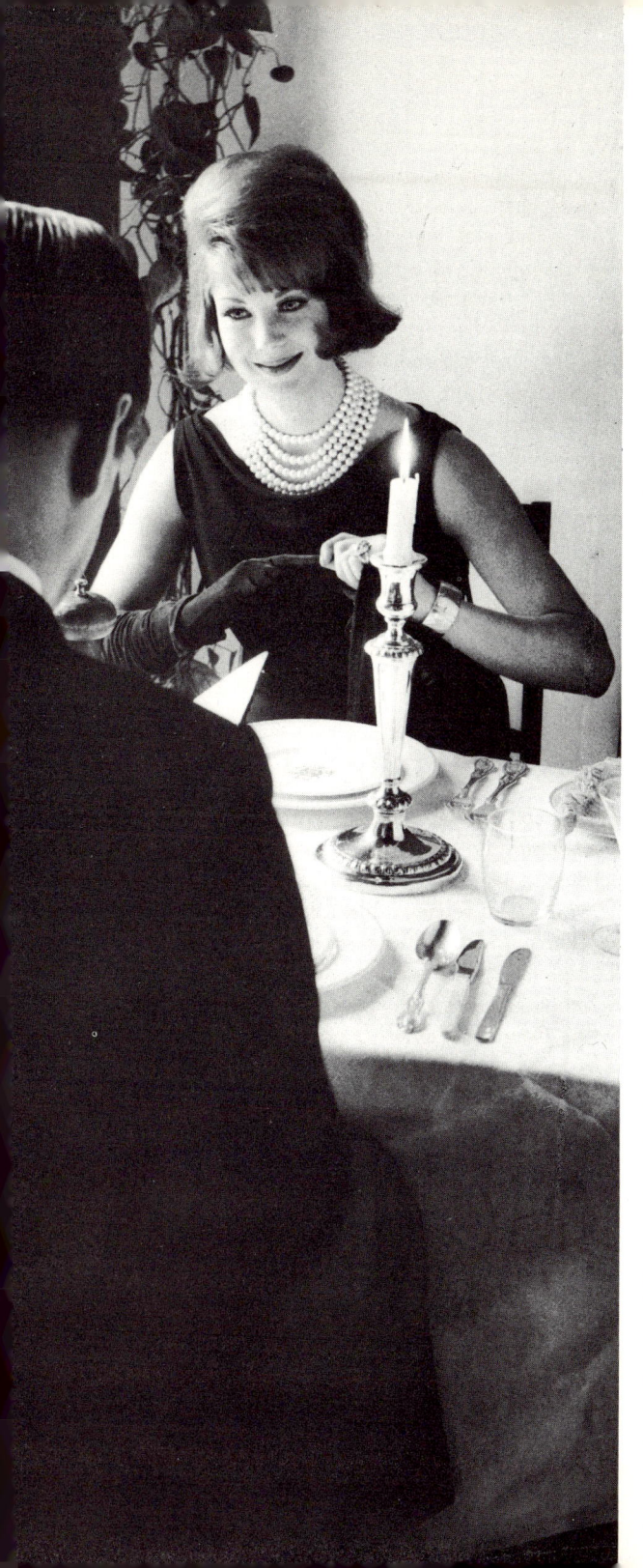

Accept his apology pleasantly—don't ask questions about it.

going to a restaurant

Let your escort lead you to his chosen place. Let him open doors for you, close doors for you, and don't try to help; leave it all to him, he is adoring every moment.

Should the head waiter come along to lead you to a table, then you both follow behind the waiter, the escort a little behind you if necessary.

When the head waiter deferentially draws back a chair, move into the seat in your most poised and queenly manner. And if the seat isn't just where you want it, then for goodness' sake wait until the waiter is out of sight before you make adjustments.

the menu

Avoid getting engrossed in conversation until the menu is settled. Your escort and the waiter may both get infuriated if the menu can't be decided because you can't stop talking.

The nicest arrangement is for your escort solicitously to discuss with you your choice and then for him to give your order and his own to the waiter—but don't worry if it doesn't work out this way. If your French or your Italian, or Greek or what have you, doesn't give you a clue to interpreting the menu, then just ask the waiter about it. It is his job to be able to tell you about everything listed. In the same way the wine waiter can be asked about choosing the appropriate wine, but all this is mainly a matter for your escort.

handbag and gloves

While the menu is being settled, you should be elegantly removing your gloves and deciding where you are going to put them and your handbag. Don't put them *on the table* because they will clutter it up and spoil its arrangement. In addition, you risk their getting spoiled by food crumbs. And don't put them *on the floor*. At some point you may desperately need your handkerchief (suppose you sneeze, or what about that tickle at the end of the nose?), and if your bag has inadvertently been kicked *under* the table, then your escort would be quite embarrassed to see you disappear from sight groping under the table.

Put handbag and gloves together on an unused chair at the table, on a window ledge, or on an under-table ledge, but if none of these is available, then put them on your lap with your table napkin on top.

table napkin or dinner napkin

This should not be folded up at the end of the meal, but just dropped down on the table as you rise.

things that may fall to the floor

As a matter of fact, at no time should your escort see you picking up articles from the floor. If a spoon, fork, or napkin has fallen, then it is really up to the waiter or waitress to retrieve this, take it away, and bring you another one (on the assumption, of course, that it is no longer clean enough for you to use, and rightly so).

Supposing, however, your bracelet has slipped quietly to the floor, and only you are aware of this. Are you then to stoop down and pick it up? Certainly not. Try looking feminine and helpless at your escort, saying, "Oh dear!... I'm afraid I've dropped my..." And before you've finished your sentence, he will, I assure you, be out of his seat and picking up the article.

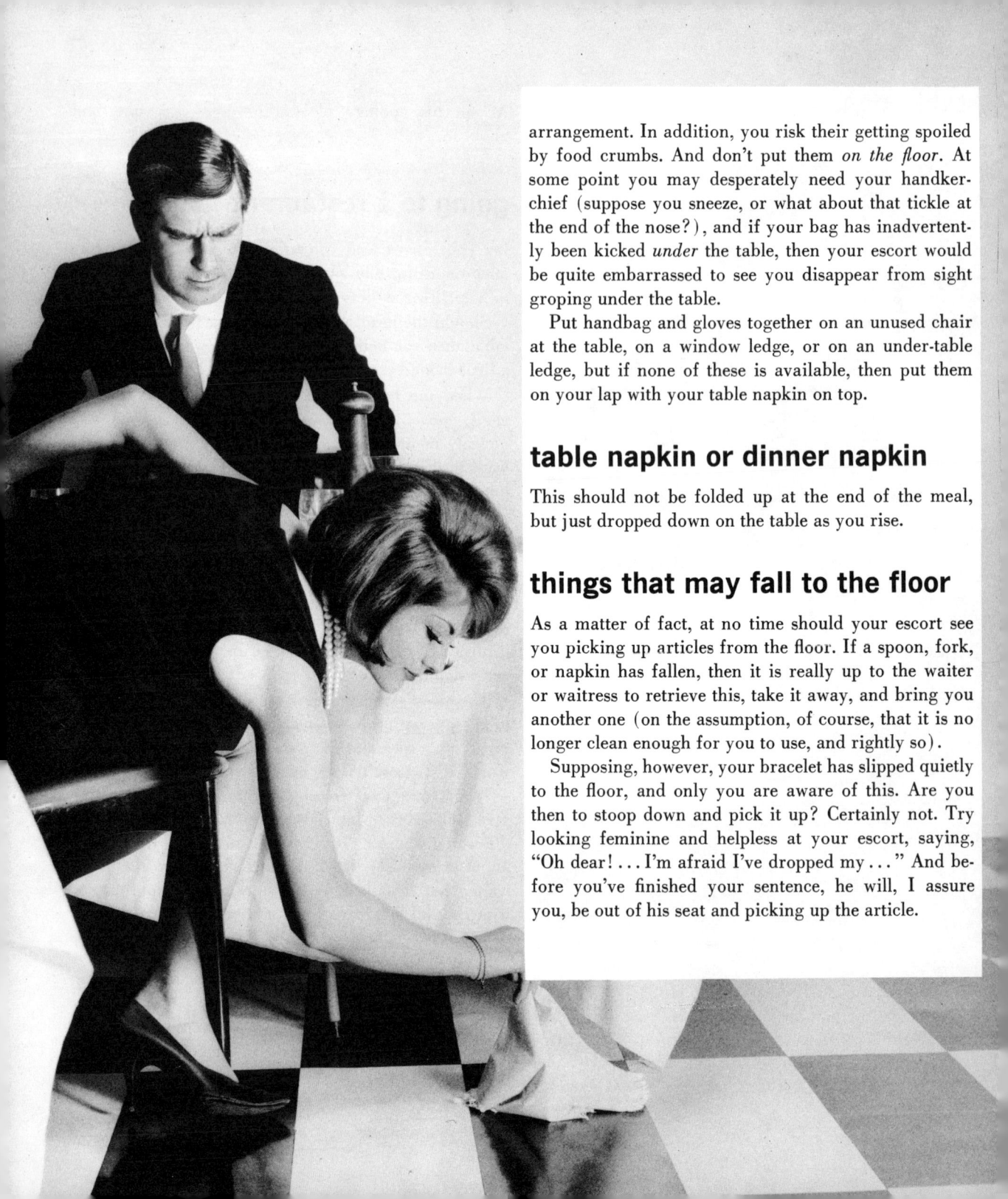

table posture

Hold yourself in good posture while at table. Nothing makes a more deplorable picture than seeing on the other side of the table someone bent double over a plate taking up food as though she has starved for a week.

conversation

This should be well balanced with the eating. Nothing is more embarrassing than finding you are left with a plateful of food when others have finished and the waiter is poised with the next course. Should *you* notice that your escort is doing just this, then you could tactfully take over the talking, or delay finishing your own plate.

the slow eater

If this applies to you, then avoid large helpings, second helpings, and things which are difficult to eat.

not sure of the correct way to eat an item on the menu

Then for goodness' sake, don't choose it. Find out for another time; or if others choose it, notice what they do, and thus build up your knowledge.

Should you be confronted with a dish which is new to you and you feel unsure about how to eat it, then try stalling by carrying on a conversation until you can pick up a clue from others. If this isn't practicable, then go ahead and eat it in the way that seems most sensible.

With regard to poultry and game, there are varying opinions as to whether it is ever correct to lift a bone with the fingers. Some authorities say definitely that it is not done. Others insist that it is. My advice would be to do it only if you are sure you can do it so naturally and fastidiously that no one could find it objectionable or unfeminine. This would preclude the greasy or otherwise difficult bone. A vegetarian like myself would of course in any case find the spectacle unattractive. My final word over this, or over many another disputed custom, is to remember that it is not always what you do that matters, but how you do it.

your finished plate

Don't just push it anywhere away from you. Leave it where it is for the waiter to collect. If he's delayed and you need the position, then move the used plate neatly to your left on the table.

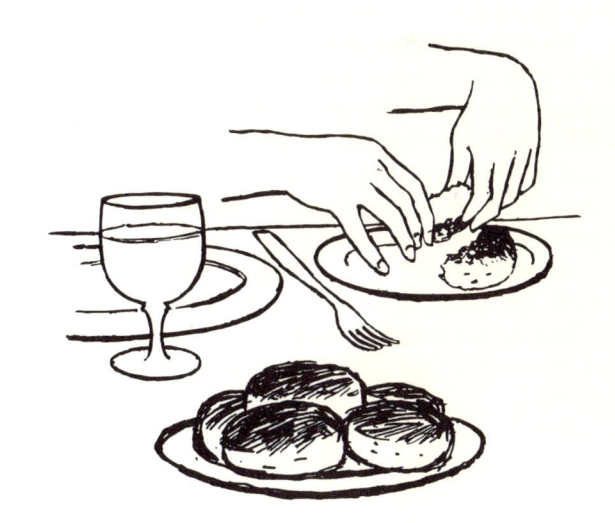

dry bread or rolls

These, of course, should be on the small plate to your left. Break down the bread or roll only sufficiently to take the small piece you need immediately, and convey this to the mouth with the fingers. (The situation is quite different when you have a *buttered* bread or roll; then you should bite off the piece needed.)

knives, forks, spoons, etc.

You will find in the place or cover in front of you, forks to the left, knives to the right, the soup spoon being at the right-hand side outside the knives. Since the soup spoon is one of the first things you are likely to use, then finding it there will remind you (in case you have forgotten) that you work through the cutlery using the outer ones first. (This would be important to remember at a private dinner or function. In a restaurant, very often, the cutlery is brought with each dish.)

the handling of the cutlery

Move the soup spoon away from you to gather the soup and take only the amount you can drink in one sip. Drink from the side of the spoon.

Don't hold knives and forks as you would pencils, but keep the handles within the palms of the hands, manipulating with the thumb and the first two fingers. Hold them slanting downwards as much as possible, and never be tempted to explain or demonstrate anything with them. Don't cut up all the food on your plate before starting to eat it.

Knife and fork (and this applies to dessert spoon and fork too) placed in a V on your plate spell to the waiter "Resting, not finished" (and rest you should from time to time, otherwise, once again, it may look as if you're starving).

The knife and fork on your plate upturned and together spell to the waiter, "Finished, please take away."

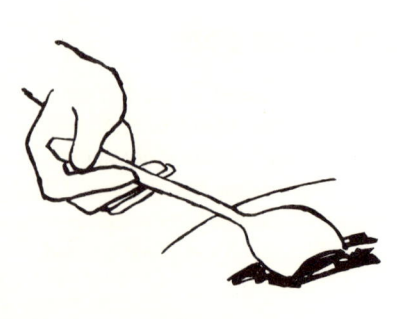

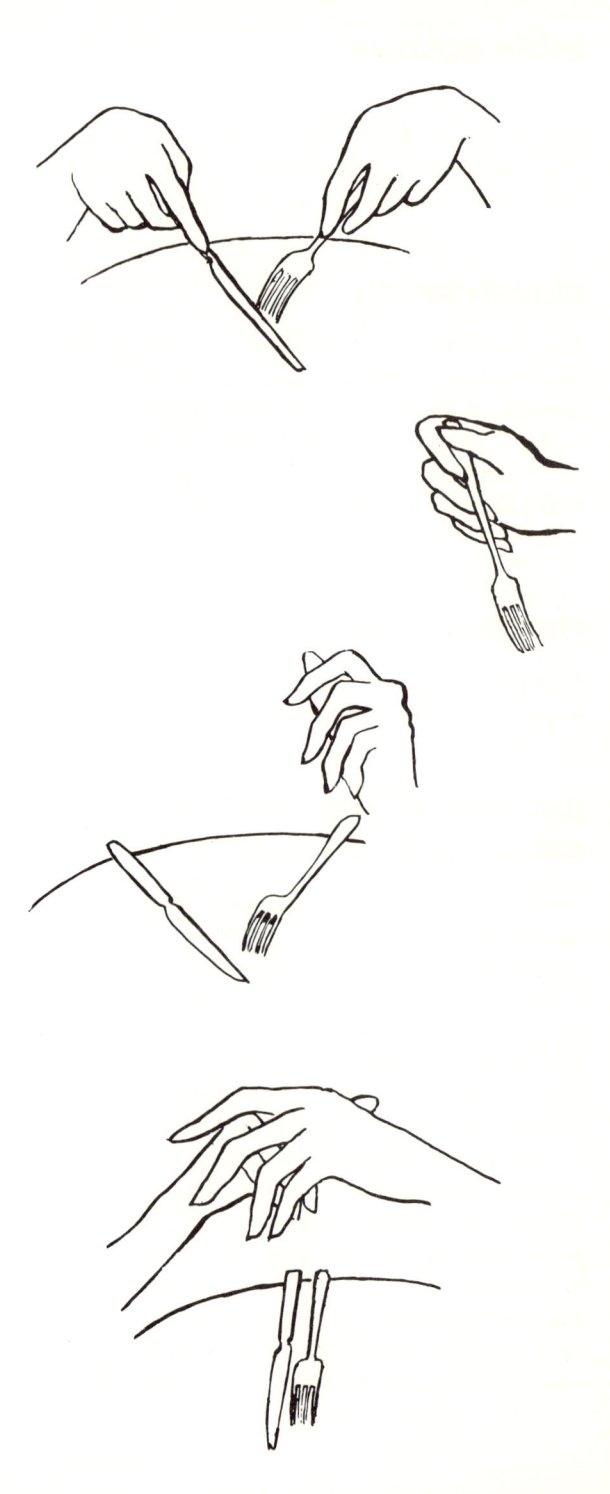

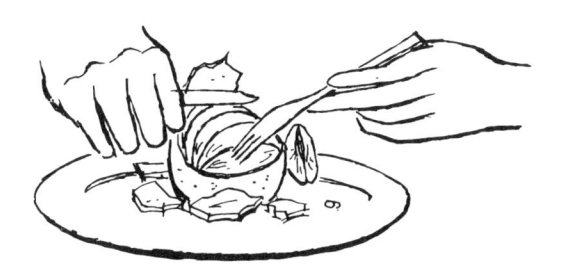

fresh fruit for dessert

Use dessert knife and fork, or just dessert knife and fingers. Quarter down as much as you can. Stones and pips should be removed from the mouth with your fingers as unobtrusively as possible, but in a perfectly natural manner. Oranges should have the skin first cut through in sections. Remove the peel and then break down the orange into its smallest sections, trying not to puncture the delicate inner skin. Put the complete small unpunctured section into your mouth and thus no juice will escape.

For apples, pears, peaches, etc., use the fruit knife and fork. Cut down to quarters or to eighths if necessary. Peel each small section and eat with the fork. If you prefer to eat the peel, then of course don't remove it. (With many fruits, and vegetables, too, for that matter, the goodness is considered to lie next to the skin.)

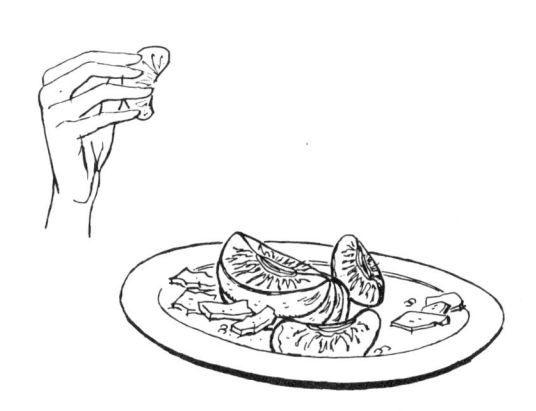

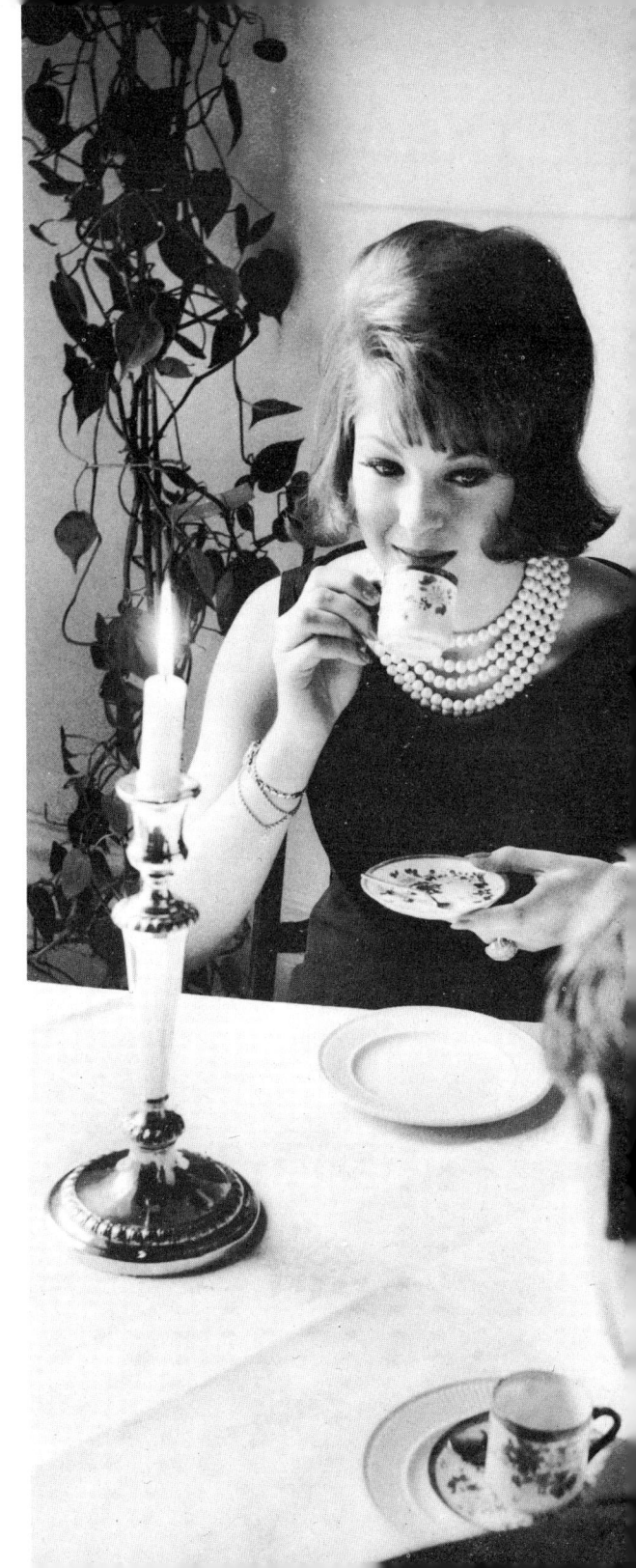

TABOOS

To round all this off, here is my ABSOLUTELY TABOO list, and I'm sure you are not guilty of any of these:

Eating with the lips apart.

Taking a second mouthful before the one in the mouth is finished.

Sipping a drink while there is still food in the mouth.

Making any noise when drinking.

Making too much noise when eating.

Taking from a main dish straight to the mouth. (This would include sandwiches, biscuits, and bread and butter.) It can look rather like communal feeding, especially if one or two others are doing it at the same time as you are. It can easily be avoided, even at a stand-up cocktail party, by pausing for a few seconds before eating.

Sprinkling salt or sugar over your own food with a serving spoon. This can be avoided by taking the required small helping on to the side of the plate, and returning the serving spoon to its dish. Of course, this doesn't apply where there is a sprinkler

Taking such large mouthfuls of food that you are unable to answer questions for an embarrassing few seconds.

Keeping dishes closely surrounding your plate instead of moving them away, or passing them on, after use.

Speaking of illness, diet, or dentistry at meals.

Leaving a spoon in a cup after stirring.

Rattling lumps of sugar around in a cup while stirring.

Eating anything with the knife.

Making up, combing hair, or picking teeth at table or in public. The right thing to do is to wait until you can go to a powder room for these operations

etiquette and behavior 83

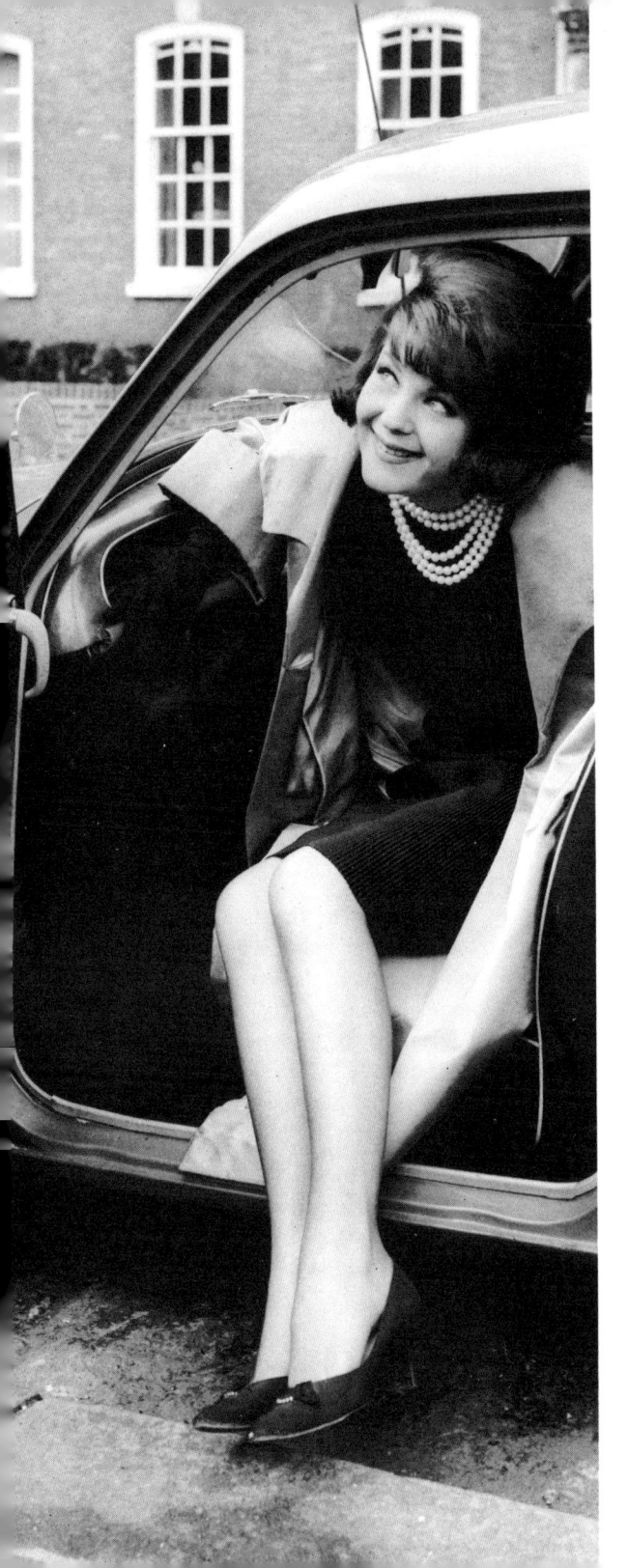

Things to leave to your escort

paying and tipping

Your escort wouldn't have asked you out unless he was prepared to undertake the paying and tipping. You'll only embarrass him (or even annoy him) by offering to share expense. Of course, should you meet a friend of the opposite sex by chance when traveling or eating out, you should then insist upon paying your own bill.

opening and closing doors

Your escort can't of course do this for you if you're always rushing through doors. On the other hand if these little courtesies never seem to occur to him, you can train him (without his realizing it) by slowing down your steps when you are both approaching a door so that he is automatically there first and opens it. You sail through with a murmured thank you under your breath, leaving him to close it.

getting into a cab

You should get into a cab first, moving to the farther side of the seat so that your escort doesn't have to scramble over your feet. Allow him to give all the instructions to the driver. When getting out, allow him to go first so that he is there to help you down. And finally, of course, allow him to pay and tip the driver.

getting out of his car

If an escort gives you a lift, then upon arrival he may wish to get out of the driving seat, to walk around, and open the car door for you from the outside. This might indeed be rare, but for goodness' sake let him do it or maybe he'll feel frustrated. If you're not sure whether he wishes to do this or not, then give him the opportunity by doodling with your handbag or gloves for a few seconds. In any case, before getting out yourself, give him the opportunity of making some gesture to open the door for you.

other vehicles

The same order applies to getting in and out of other vehicles. How often on a bus has one seen the young man getting up and standing back so that his girl friend can go first to get off. One can almost feel his thought that he *knows* he is doing the right thing—Ladies first. The only way you can train him here would be to murmur, "No, *you* go first, and then you'll be there to catch me if I fall."

holding your elbow protectively in crowds

This is quite correct. But don't let the escort hold your arm all the time in the street. This can look sloppy and in any case, neither of you can thus execute good deportment. Incidentally, if you ever hold his arm, never let him feel you're a ton weight. He should only be aware of the most ethereal being lightly poised at his side. And never be seen with your hand resting on the escort's arm while he stalks along with both hands in his pockets. He may not mean it, but it gives the impression that he couldn't care less.

helping you off and on with a coat

carrying your case or parcels

picking up any dropped articles

Graciously accept all such little courtesies with a thank you or just with a rewarding smile.

Introductions

when making them

If you tend to get embarrassed and to forget names, then try to think ten seconds ahead and get your facts right. The two people being introduced are probably not criticizing you at this moment. Their interest is sure to be concentrated upon the other person. Speak clearly and slowly. Make it a gracious moment. Introduce a man *to* a woman—but common sense would dictate to you that when, say, introducing a 16-year-old girl friend to your grandfather, then the honor would be due to your grandfather by virtue of his age. When introducing a friend to your parents, introduce him or her to your mother first, then to your father. Between women, the honor is due to the married woman, or the older woman, whichever your tact suggests.

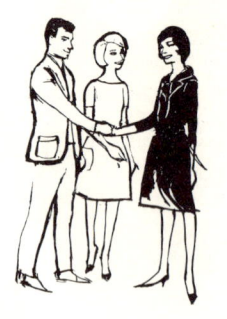

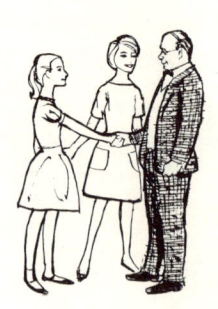

Similarly, between men, the honor is due to the married man or the older man. A good plan is to train yourself to *look at*, or take the other person *to* the one to whom the honor is due.

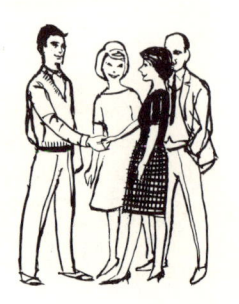

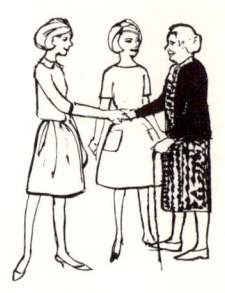

The simple forms of expression used nowadays are, "I want to introduce..., May I introduce...?, Let me introduce...." When you have finished the introduction, then it's quite the nicest thing you can do to mention something that the two have in common, or mention their interests. This should start them off naturally in conversation with each other, which is distinctly useful if you are a hostess and wish to slip away to attend to other matters.

when being introduced

Train yourself to listen for the name and remember it. However, nobody really minds if you didn't catch the name (the fault may lie in the manner in which the introduction was made). You can always say afterwards, "I'm sorry, I didn't catch your name," which gives you both the opportunity of reaffirming names. If you try to use the new name over and over again in conversation during the next few minutes this might help you remember it.

Smoking

if you don't

Just say, "No, thank you," and don't give any explanations other than, "I don't smoke." This may prevent the cigarettes from being offered again. Don't make a sudden decision in public to smoke for the first time ever. You've all seen the spectacle in a film or play when the young heroine does just this in an impetuous attempt to appear sophisticated, instead of which, she gets smoke in her eyes, splutters, and generally just doesn't know how to manage.

if you must

When you have accepted a cigarette, don't just go wandering around doing nothing further about it. Usually the cigarette is followed up by the offer of a light, which should be graciously and femininely accepted. Rolling a cigarette around your lips to moisten it looks frightful. One simple moistening of the lips is quite sufficient, and this should be done quite unnoticeably.

Remember, too, that it looks unattractive and unfeminine to leave a cigarette in your mouth while speaking, or to flick cigarette ash all over the place.

The use of a cigarette holder while smoking lends a certain air of sophistication which needs living up to (rather in the same way as when wearing a hat veil or carrying a long, slim umbrella). Use a holder with an ejector to save that poking and prying about to remove the cigarette stub.

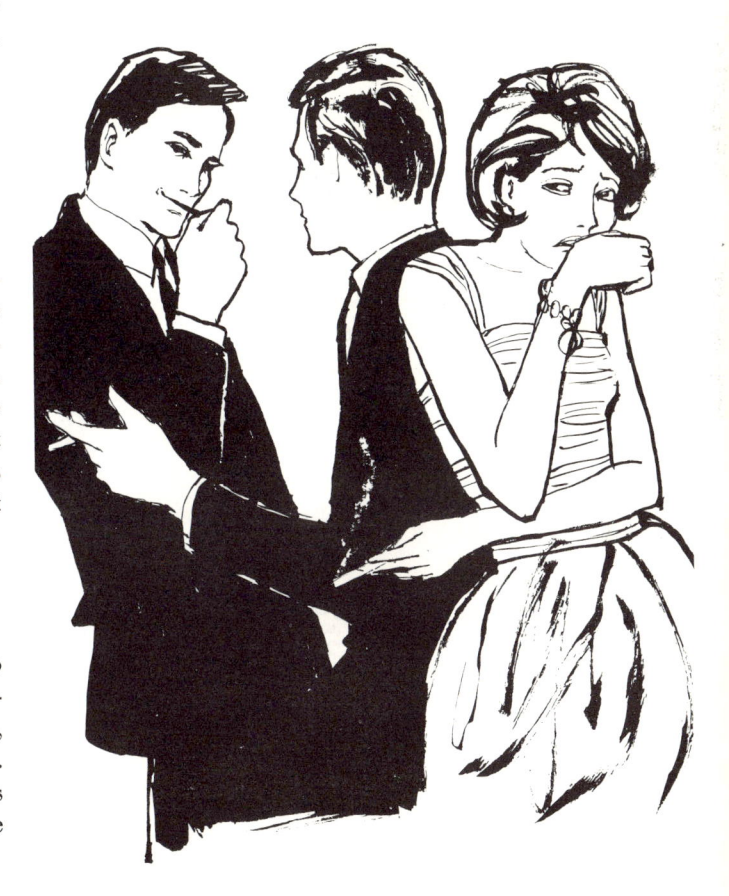

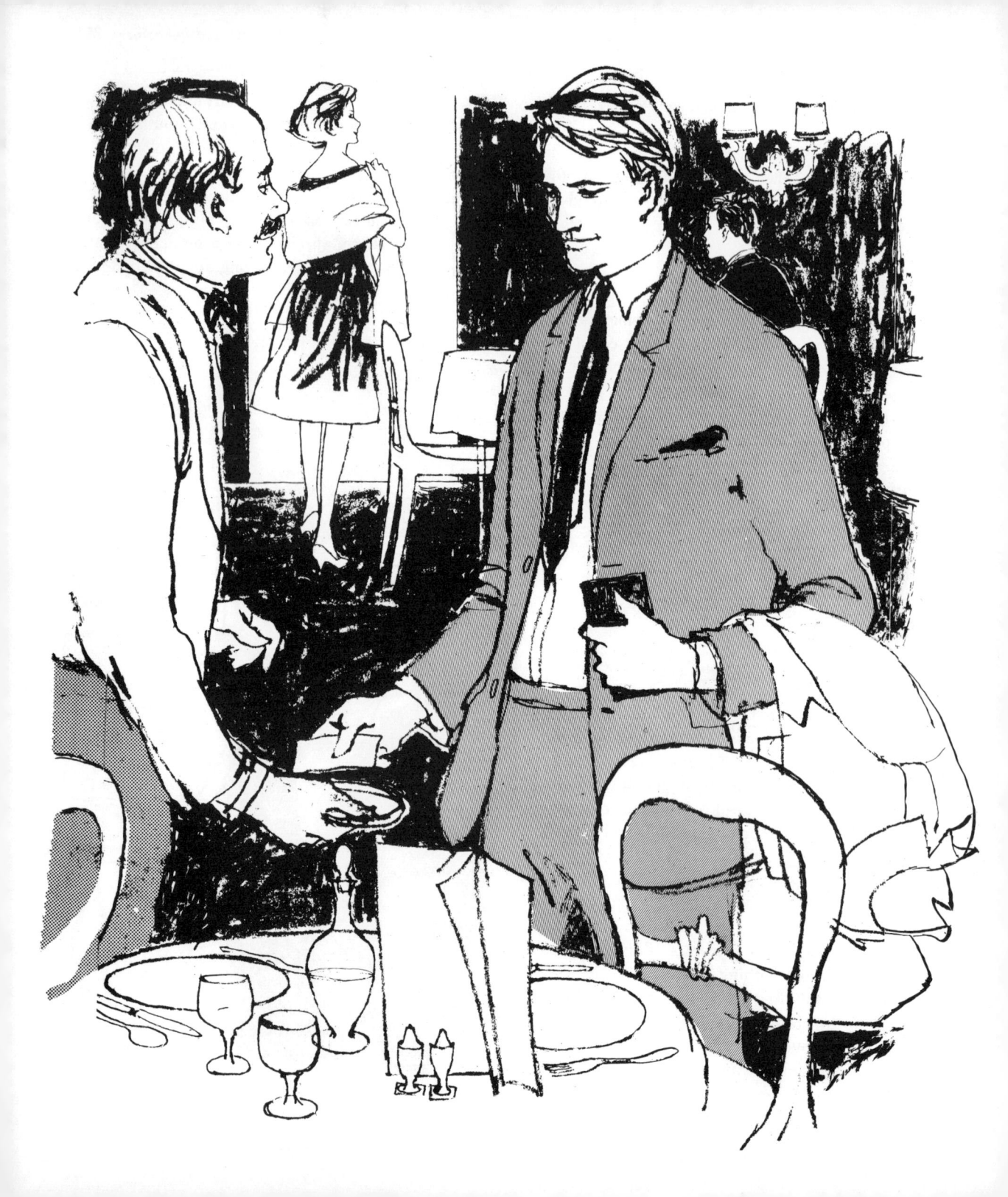

etiquette and behavior 87

Tipping

The two golden rules to guide you when tipping are (*a*) base the amount of the tip upon ten to fifteen per cent of the bill and (*b*) never tip the proprietor or manager.

Try to make your expression of personal appreciation the important thing, and be casual and unobtrusive about the money. Decide yourself how much tip you will give.

Hotels

Be as courteous and considerate as if you were accepting hospitality in a friend's house.

Leave your luggage to be brought in by the hotel staff, and relinquish hand lugage at the entrance, keeping only your handbag.

Go straight to the reception desk upon arrival and claim your room, or book a room, and sign the visitors' book. Then allow yourself to be shown to your room. Do not linger in the hall or lounge before doing this. For one thing, you should be in your room to receive your luggage, and of course to give a small tip to whoever brings it.

During a short stay most of your tipping can be left until departure. During a long stay, it is best to tip after the first day or so, particularly the head porter, the head waiter, and your table waiter, then again halfway through and upon departure. But all this is entirely at your discretion. If you are expecting visitors, leave word at the reception desk where you are to be found in the hotel.

Ask for your bill well in advance of your departure. Allow about ten per cent to cover all final tips.

At some resort hotels nowadays a charge of ten per cent is automatically added to the bill to cover all tips.

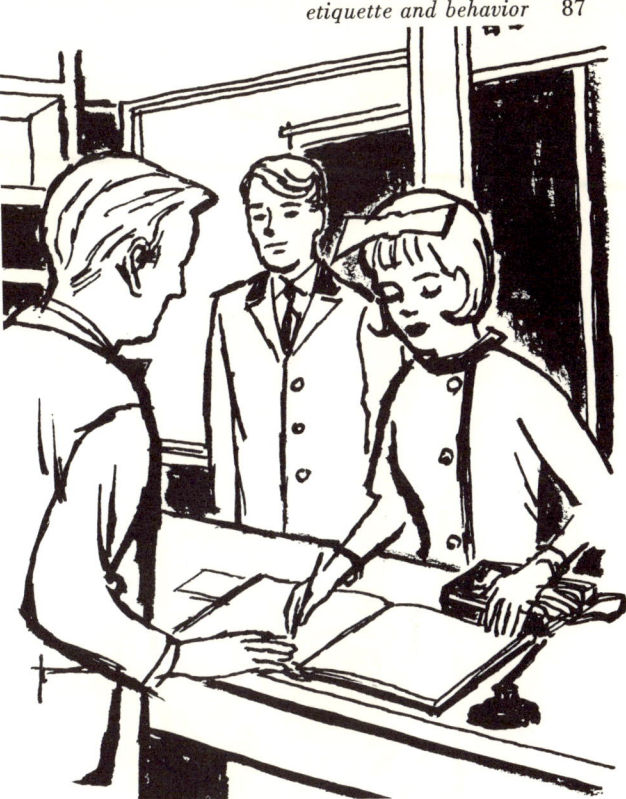

If this is the case you will probably find a card in your room which says so.

A few precious hints

your front door

Never close it until your guests have disappeared from sight. If you do, even if you don't mean it, it gives the impression you are glad to see them go.

leaving doors and windows open

You may not mind rattling windows, flapping curtains, banging doors, and drafts all around the house, not to mention sitting in a room with no sense of privacy or quiet; but *probably other people do*, and no member of a family and certainly no hostess can afford to ignore these things.

arguing

Never allow yourself to get nettled or to shout down anyone. Rather take the viewpoint of the man who said: "I heartily disagree with you, but would defend to the hilt your right to express your opinion." Or the whole thing is expressed rather nicely in the well-known French saying, *Chacun à son goût.* And of course, never argue the point with perfect strangers at a place of entertainment over such matters as noise or the wearing of a hat that obscures your view. If a polite request such as: "I'm sure you don't realize it, but your conversation (or your hat, etc., as the case may be) is . . ." If this approach doesn't achieve the desired result, then the matter should be referred to an usher to be dealt with by the management.

restroom and bathroom

Never fail to indicate to guests where these are. The right moment for this may arise upon arrival, after a meal, or when they are getting ready to leave.

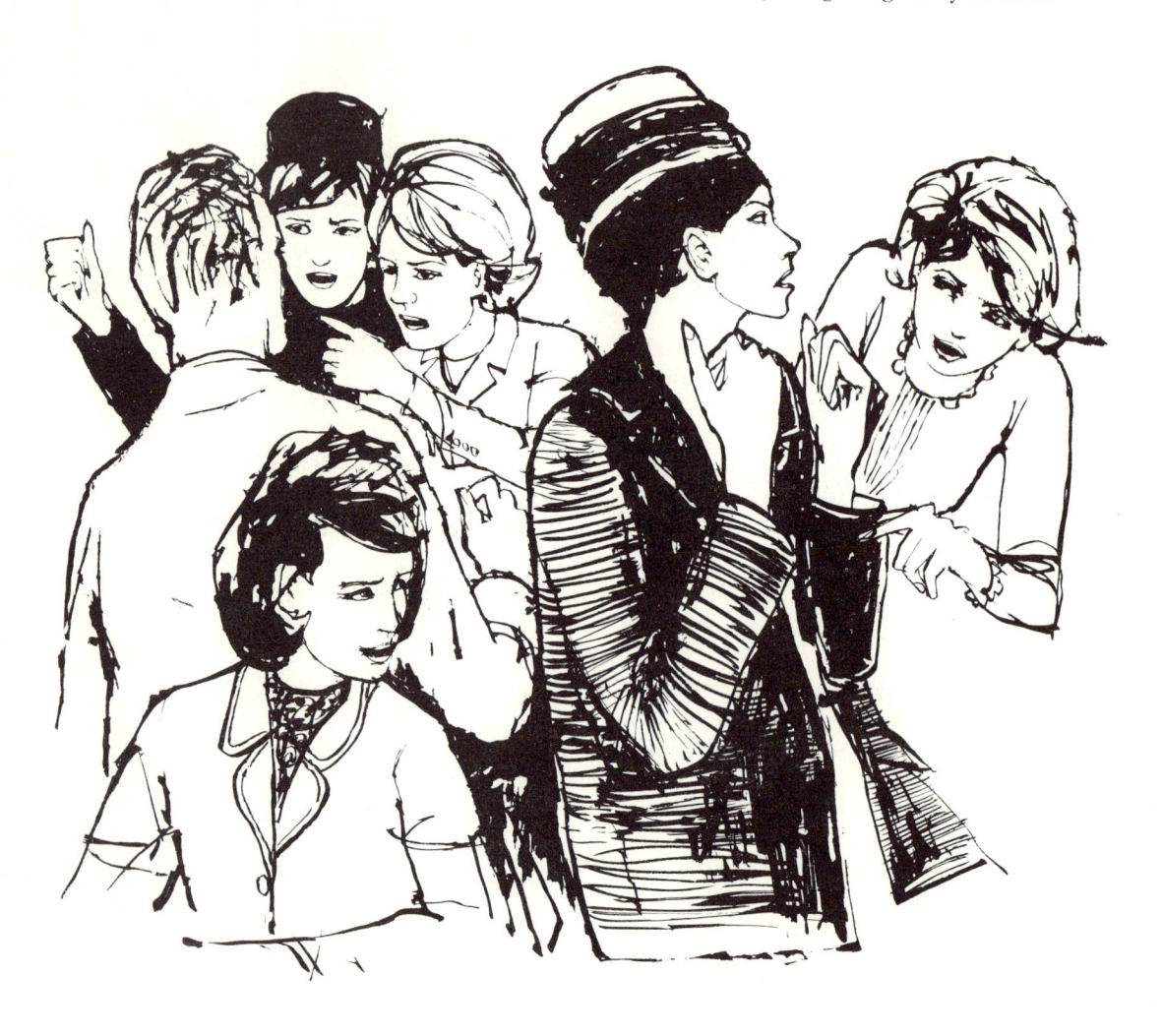

11 interviews

These are frequently milestones in your life. Therefore it is worth while planning your own very private minor campaign to insure that you do yourself justice. Practically everything I have dealt with in the earlier chapters has some bearing on success at an interview, but let us check through the most important points:

dress

To meet the occasion, this should be neat, quiet, and in the best of taste, with impeccable accessories (plain shoes, fresh gloves, and handbag; spotless inside and out). A hat can help to give you confidence and is useful to keep control of your hair if the weather is blowy or bad; but don't wear one if you're not used to it, because you might feel awkward.

grooming

Naturally you will be as fresh as a daisy with beautifully cared for hands and shining hair.

makeup

Makeup should be just right, not too much, but enough to make you feel that you are looking your best.

getting there

If you're a wise girl, you will have looked up the address on your street map and found out about traveling arrangements *days beforehand*. Allow about twice the time you think you will need to get there so that the entire journey can be conducted in a calm and unhurried frame of mind. **You will not do your best if you arrive hurried, blown, and breathless.**

arriving

Walk slowly into the building—and get the feel of it. Be ready to say "Good morning" (with a smile) to everyone, starting with the elevator attendant and the person at the reception desk. Give your name, the time of your appointment, and the name of the person you have come to see.

butterflies in the tummy

The best way to avoid this and to keep cool and calm is to indulge in as much conscious deep breathing as possible, from the moment of getting out of bed right up to the interview. If you can, walk the last few blocks or so to the interview, breathing deeply and rhythmically. After the interview you will probably realize that the butterflies were quite unnecessary, that everyone was friendly and helpful. And, what is more, after every interview, you will feel that you have grown a little....

At the interview

This is where spontaneity should be allowed to take over, and you must be sincere and natural. It is not the moment for thinking too hard about training and techniques. If you haven't by now trained yourself to walk well, make a good entrance, smile at people, sit down gracefully, control your mannerisms, then this is *not the moment to start practicing.*

A prospective employer isn't only interested in your ability and qualifications for the job, but also in your personality and character. These are usually quite as important to him as efficiency. Prepare ahead your replies to the likely questions.

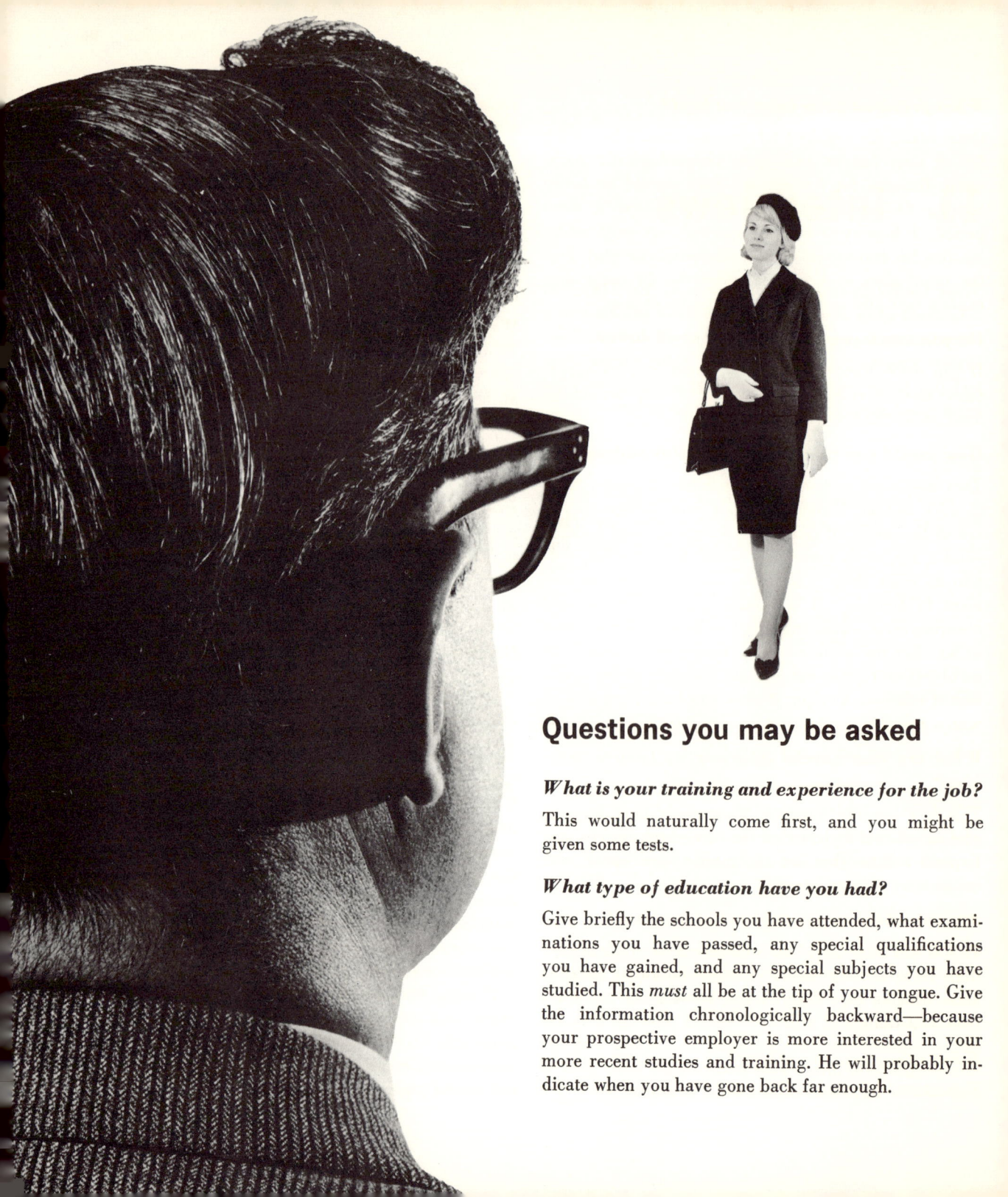

Questions you may be asked

What is your training and experience for the job?
This would naturally come first, and you might be given some tests.

What type of education have you had?
Give briefly the schools you have attended, what examinations you have passed, any special qualifications you have gained, and any special subjects you have studied. This *must* all be at the tip of your tongue. Give the information chronologically backward—because your prospective employer is more interested in your more recent studies and training. He will probably indicate when you have gone back far enough.

What previous posts have you held?

Once again, the required information should be on the tip of your tongue and given chronologically backward. Reasons for leaving any jobs should be forthcoming. If you have had several jobs over a short period, I hope you will have some very convincing reasons for leaving each one, otherwise you may give the impression of being irresponsible. In particular, explain *why* you wish to leave your present post.

Do you think you would like to work here?

If you really want the job, here would be your opportunity to show enthusiasm. Find out all you can beforehand about the firm and its work.

How would you travel to work at this address?

They may want to assess the possibility of your getting to work on time. Should you come from a distance, you are at the mercy of public transportation and weather (and a fog could mean you would be hours late). If you do come from a distance, this would be the moment to mention (if it should apply) that the best morning train would only get you to work ten minutes or so after the required time. There will probably be no objection to this, but you put yourself on the wrong foot if you only mention it after you have started work with a new firm.

What are your special interests, or leisure activities?

This is a favorite question. Your reply here helps to give an all-round picture of the sort of person you are. Expand a little (but not too much), and speak with enthusiasm of your interests.

Are you about to get engaged or married?

This is not necessarily an impertinent or prying question. There could be many reasons why a firm needs to know whether they could be sure of your services for a reasonable length of time.

What salary are you asking?

Sometimes, of course, the salary is stated when the vacancy is advertised. If not, you will appear to be most unbusinesslike if you have no idea how much to ask for. Think this well out ahead.

We have decided that you are the person we are looking for, and we are offering you the job.

By now you should have formed some idea whether it's *your* job. If you're one hundred per cent sure, then accept. If you're not, then say you wish to think it over or discuss it with your parents and would like to let them know in the morning. No one will think any the less of you for wanting to give the matter some thought. As a matter of fact, it would be no good to them, or to you, if you made a hurried decision and then found out after you'd been working there a few days that it was a mistake.

How soon can you start?

If it's your first job, then give yourself a few days' breather. If you're already working, then say that you must give so much notice and you could only start on such a day—give the date and day if possible.

Couldn't you possibly start sooner than that?

There could be more behind this question than you realize. If you're obviously prepared to walk out on your present post (perhaps over-anxious not to lose the new opportunity), then you will give the impression of being unreliable. It would be best to offer to find out from your present employers whether they would be prepared to meet you on the question of notice. When you return to your present employers, seek out an executive and *put all your cards on the table*. Say how much the new offer means to your career and how grateful you would be if they could release you sooner than the due date (and be sure to say how happy you have been working for them).

Perhaps five years later at some vital point in your career you will be asked to give the names of all the firms you have worked for, and quite apart from the principle of the thing, you will be so glad that you have left a good trail behind you.

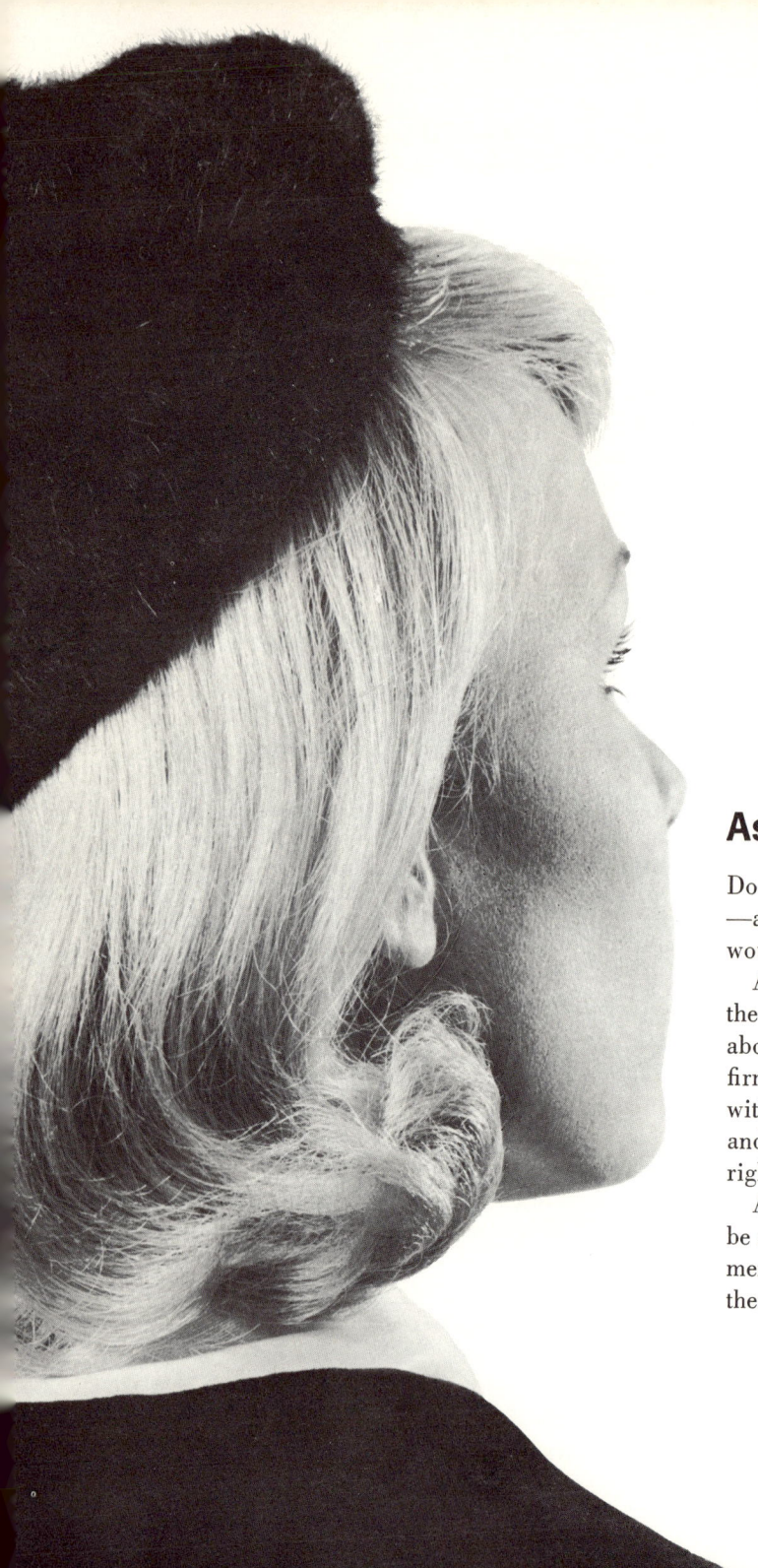

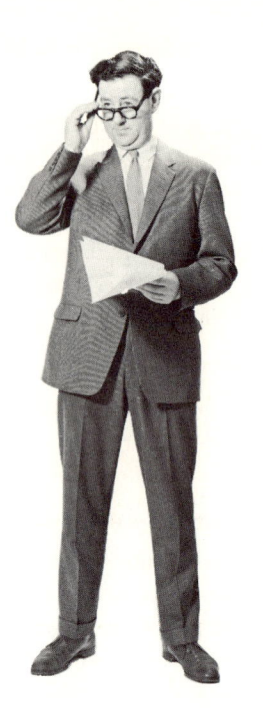

Ask questions yourself

Do not hesitate to ask questions yourself about the job —and show keen interest in exactly what work you would be doing.

At the end of the interview, if you have been offered the job, ask very politely about the hours, particularly about the lunch time. (I mention this because some firms are apt to let the lunch time get swallowed up with urgent work rather too often, and psychologically and for your health's sake, it is a good thing to get right away from your place of business at midday.)

Ask too about the vacation arrangements. Should you be already committed to some vacation, then be sure to mention it, and see what they say. If it is imminent, then offer to take it without pay.

12 first job

Who doesn't feel strange on the first day! But wait for the thrill of receiving your first salary.

Have you any doubts about your ability for the job? Again, who doesn't have! But remember, the firm selected *you* for the job, and therefore has confidence in you. Moreover, they know you need a little time to get used to things. Label all your doubts growing pains, and after a few weeks, when you are happily settled down, you will see that this is just what they were.

If you are wondering what to wear, follow the advice given for what to wear at an interview where it applies. In addition, avoid outfits which are sleeveless, low-cut, strong-colored, transparent, or too figure-revealing, because any of these could be an embarrassment to you and to others.

You are likely to meet many new people on your first day at work. You might even be taken on a tour of the premises and introduced to employees as you go through. However, it is obviously important to remember the names of executives and of the people you are to work with closely. If you know you are not very good at remembering names, then try to apply any little personal association that springs to your mind that will help. Here are one or two examples to show you what I mean:

Mr. Sewell...can't see well, wears glasses...

Miss Green...very keen...

Mr. Major...looks the part, or...looks a minor (as the case may be)

Mrs. Hughes...is huge, or...is not huge (as the case may be)

Mr. Johnson...bit like my uncle John...

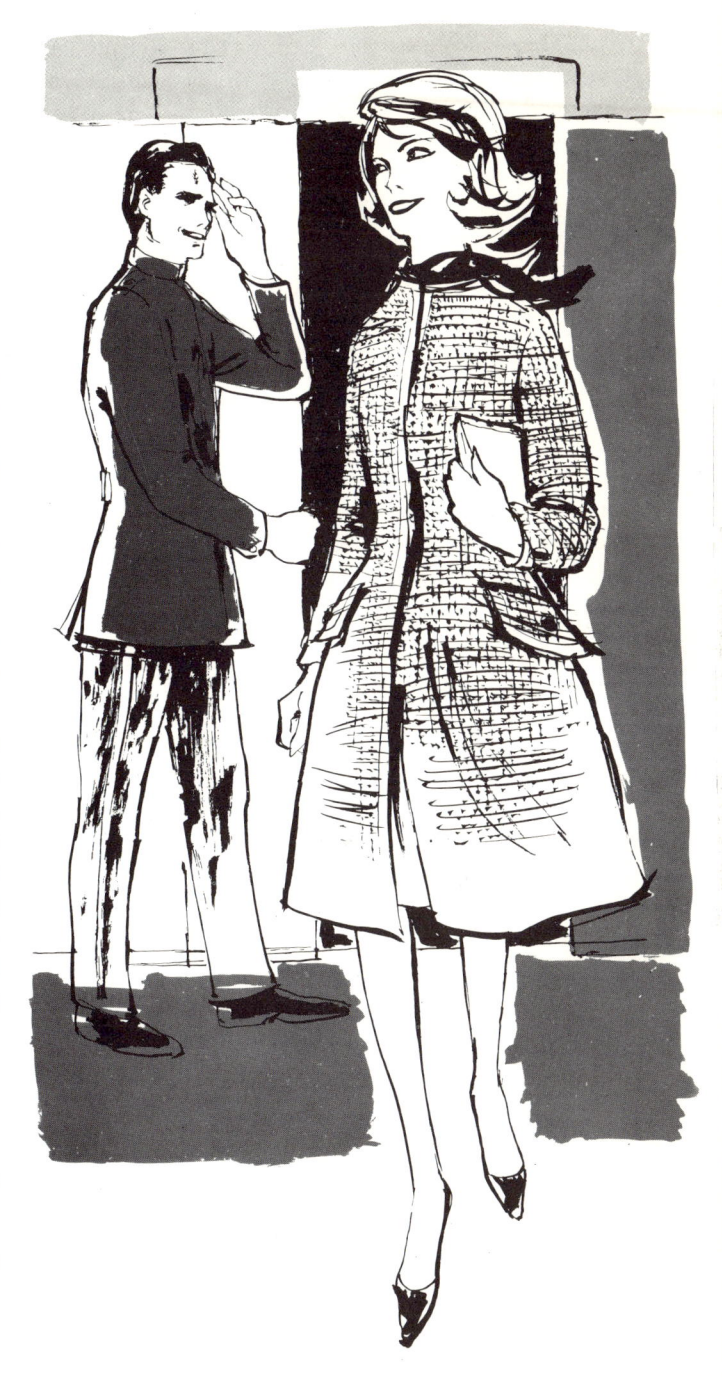

Then as soon as you have a moment to yourself (a coffee break, for instance), jot down quickly these ideas on a piece of paper which you have put ready in your handbag for just this purpose. That evening your notes will help you to visualize each person. And the following day you will be able to say: "Good morning, Mr. Sewell," "Good morning, Miss Green," etc., which will duly stagger everyone and so get you off to a flying start.

Your work may be quite clearly defined, but always offer to help someone who is temporarily swamped with work, or working on urgent work against time.

Avoid asking too many questions. Stick to those which are immediately necessary for your work.

Don't have false pride about tidying up jobs, doing errands, making coffee or tea. After all, an errand may get you out for a welcome breather, and making tea may provide an opportunity for meeting the boss.

If you happen to be with the boss when he receives a telephone call, or a visitor, then silently leave the room. (He will indicate if this is not necessary.)

In a small office you will almost certainly be required to help with the answering of the telephone, and to do as much filtering of calls as possible. Telephone technique comes within the orbit of public relations, and you may be instructed exactly how to deal with callers. In any case:

(*a*) Cultivate a pleasant, clear voice, not speaking too abruptly or too quickly. (Remember, your voice may be the first contact with a new customer.)

(*b*) If the callers have to be kept waiting, keep on returning to the phone reassuring them that you haven't forgotten them and that you are sorry to keep them waiting. Inquire whether they would prefer to hang up and call back or have you call them when their party is available.

(*c*) Be very circumspect about what you say about other members of the staff and their movements. It might not be politic, for instance, to say at 10 A.M. that a certain person hasn't arrived yet. It is better to say that a person is in or out—with no explanations.

Avoid being late either in the morning or after lunch. Get down to work as quickly as possible upon arrival. Try not to be a clock-watcher, even if you have got an exciting date at six o'clock—the time will seem to go much more quickly if you concentrate upon what you have to do.

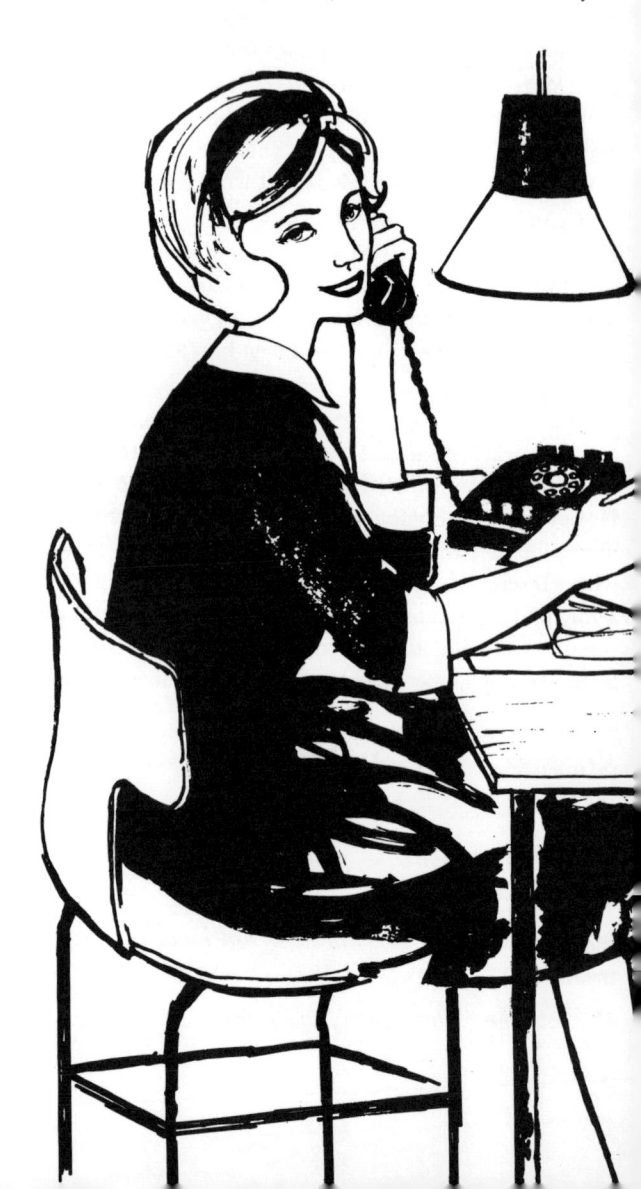

Of course, exchange friendly words with coworkers, but don't arrive at the office or your place of work with the one idea of telling everyone about the dance you have been to, the film you have seen, and so on. It is, in fact, better to err on the side of being quiet and reserved.

If you need some time off, or to leave early, use your discretion how much of the reason you offer. Usually the boss is satisfied with the explanation of urgent personal affairs, and he would be impatient of some long personal explanation. Try to avoid asking any favors until you have been with the firm some time. Moreover, in the same breath in which you ask for time off, offer to make it up some other day. This puts you on the right foot. If you have in the past willingly put in extra time when occasion demanded, then the probability is that the boss will not dream of accepting your offer. Choose the right moment, too, to ask your favor, not Monday morning (many people don't feel at their best then); not Friday (bosses are apt to be engrossed in the matter of salaries, insurance, and getting away for the weekend); not after luncheon (when the boss may have been entertaining clients and have a lot on his mind). The best times are obviously, therefore, after morning or afternoon coffee on Tuesdays, Wednesdays, or Thursdays.

You will most probably be given your own chair, desk, table, or bench in a spot to call your own. Keep these in apple-pie order and take with you on the very first day:

1 *Towel and soap in washable container.*

2 *Spare makeup in washable container.*

3 *Spare shoes and stockings. (Should you get caught in a shower, you would be most uncomfortable spending three or four hours with wet feet.)*

4 *A coat hanger.*

Of course, the more poised and charming you are the more you will be noticed by everyone—including, unfortunately, the wolves. If you haven't already got it, you will acquire a sixth sense about any undesirable approach from a member of the opposite sex. We all recognize the ladies' man—he doesn't realize it, but it is (to a woman) written all over his face. Advice:

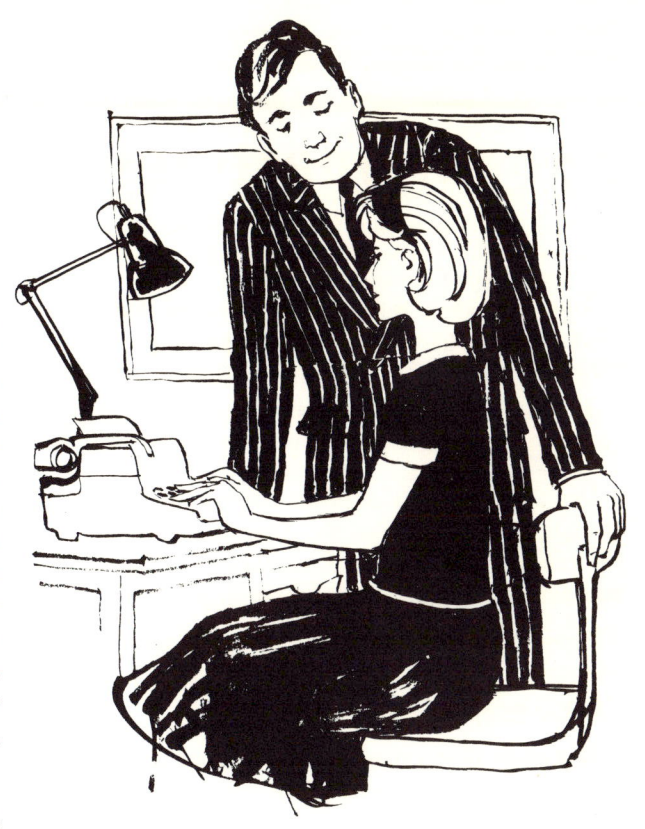

(*a*) Don't by the bat of an eyelid let him think you have noticed him. Take unobtrusive avoiding action.

(*b*) If this doesn't work, then take obtrusive avoiding action.

(*c*) Sometimes it may be necessary to arrange friendly protection from another girl on the staff who works near you.

(*d*) Maintain your reserve and dignity: these are your most effective weapons.

As a matter of fact, if there is anything at all which you find embarrassing, I advise you to discuss it with someone whom you trust.

13 an apartment of your own

I am reminded of the one young man student I once had in a group of about thirty-five young women. Whatever cropped up in his life or in class, he would remark: "Well, it's all good practice, isn't it?" An apartment of your own (and what teenager doesn't rather yearn to have one?) can be a good practice for a home of your own one day. Here are a few points to remember.

the legal aspects

These should be watertight and well understood by you. Ask the advice of someone who knows about these things.

a modern apartment

This is easier to run than an old-fashioned one.

wall-to-wall carpets everywhere

This streamlines cleaning, and makes for warmth, comfort, and quietness.

decorative effects

One or two lamp-lit corners and some plants are probably all you need—the more you have around, the more complicated is the dusting and cleaning.

organized order

In the bathroom and kitchen it is particularly necessary to put away and tidy as you go all the week. Then each weekend, or one night a week, clean *one* of your rooms very thoroughly. Thus you keep reasonable pace with things and the apartment doesn't become a burden.

doing the dishes

Always do this immediately. Use a no rinse, no wipe washing-up product and have a permanent arrangement for leaving the dishes to dry. (Dishes are the only things you should ever leave around out of place when you go out of the apartment in the morning.)

drip-dry

Organize some permanent arrangement for drip-drying so that garments can practically be washed out as taken off. (Gorgeous not to have an accumulation of washing.)

drains and sinks

Give these a regular inspection, and for goodness' sake watch what goes down the sink or you may find the waste pipe has blocked up at a most inconvenient moment.

taps

Avoid leaving them dripping for hours while you're out —or you may get landed with a drip-drip that can't be cured until you've called in the plumber for new washers.

marketing

Have one of everything *in reserve*. The moment you use the reserve, put the item down on your shopping list. Thus you should never run out of essentials.

housework and health and beauty treatment

Maybe you don't like housework. Very few of us do, but we like the result of it. The more we hate it, the

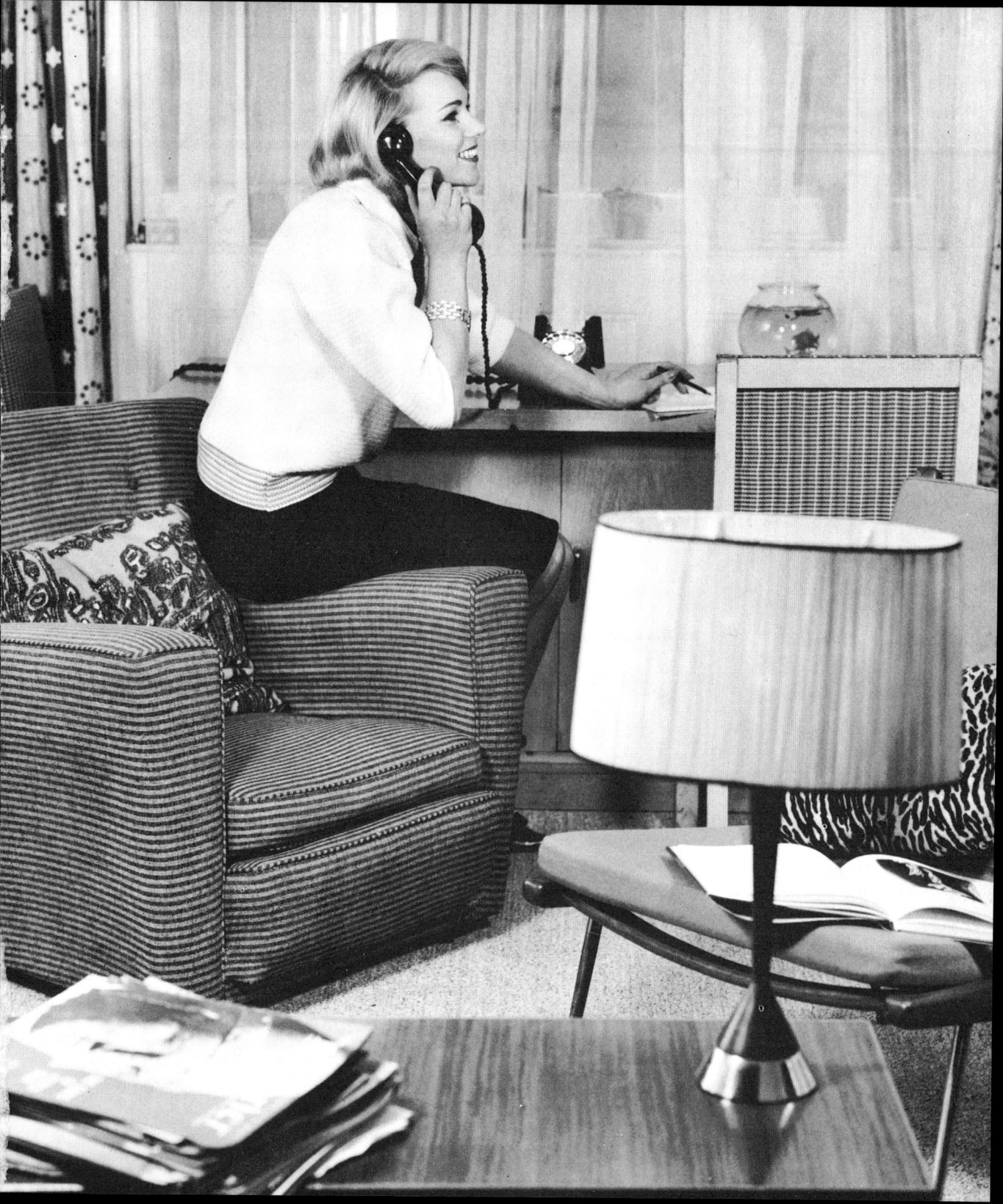

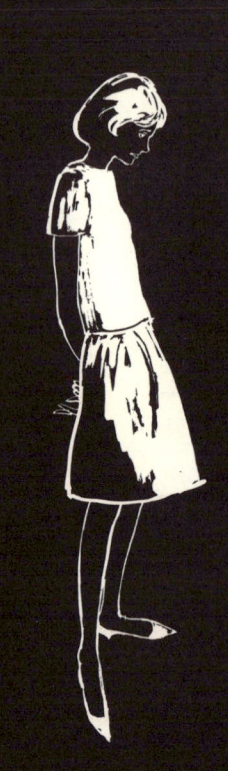

do you ever **give** *parties?*

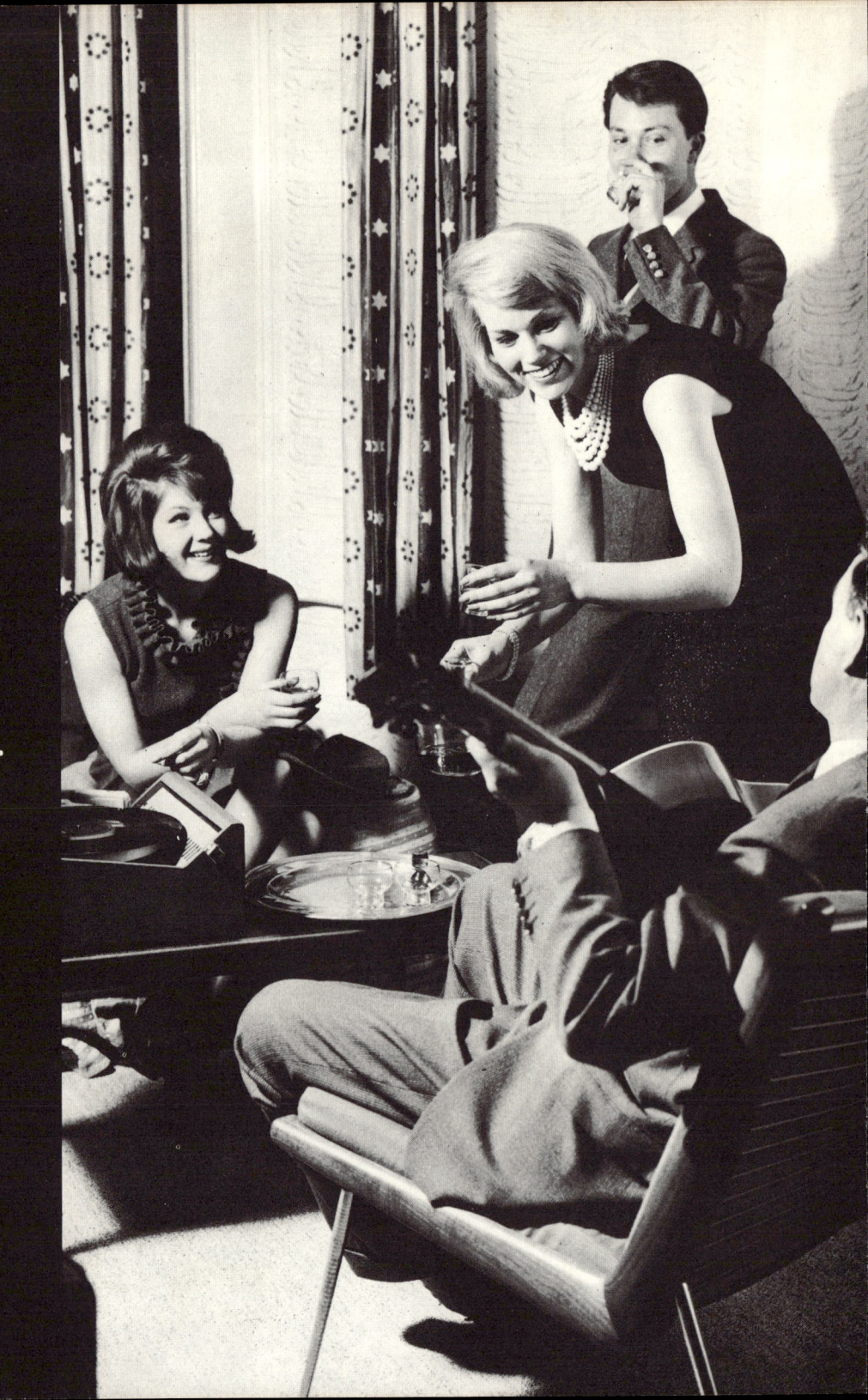

more it is necessary to do it all as though we *love it*. Otherwise we tend to rush through it at speed, ending up physically exhausted and a nervous wreck. After all, all the stretching, bending, kneeling (with tummy drawn in, of course) is wonderful exercise, and a wise girl will enjoy it as such. As with any exercise, you will find you are breathing more deeply. Therefore, open the windows and air yourself as well as the apartment.

entertaining and being entertained

It is a very different thing entertaining on your own from playing hostess in your parents' home where there is an established background and where your parents are really the hosts. And so start modestly by, say, inviting one or two girl friends in for coffee one evening. Even so, plan the refreshments, the lighting, and the music.

There was once a girl who wrote to one of the agony columns of a woman's magazine, wailing that she never got asked to parties. The cryptic reply has stuck in my mind ever since: *Do you ever give any?*

dressing table

This should always look immaculate and as expensively feminine as possible. Train yourself to keep as much as possible of your paraphernalia out of sight in closets and drawers. An armory of cosmetics in vast array on your dressing table gives the impression that your beauty only survives with the aid of these things.

keeping a nice balance

On the one hand try to leave your apartment so that you wouldn't be ashamed to take anyone back with you. (It can be a bit of a shock to a friend, and an embarrassment to you, if you return to your apartment together to find an unmade bed, clothes lying around, unwashed dishes, etc.). On the other hand—and here I will pass on to you the opinion of one of the most unforgettable characters I have met, a film critic of international repute—a perfectly kept home with not a speck of dust in sight, everything polished to the hilt and cared for, every cushion puffed up and in place, is a *sign of a misspent life*.

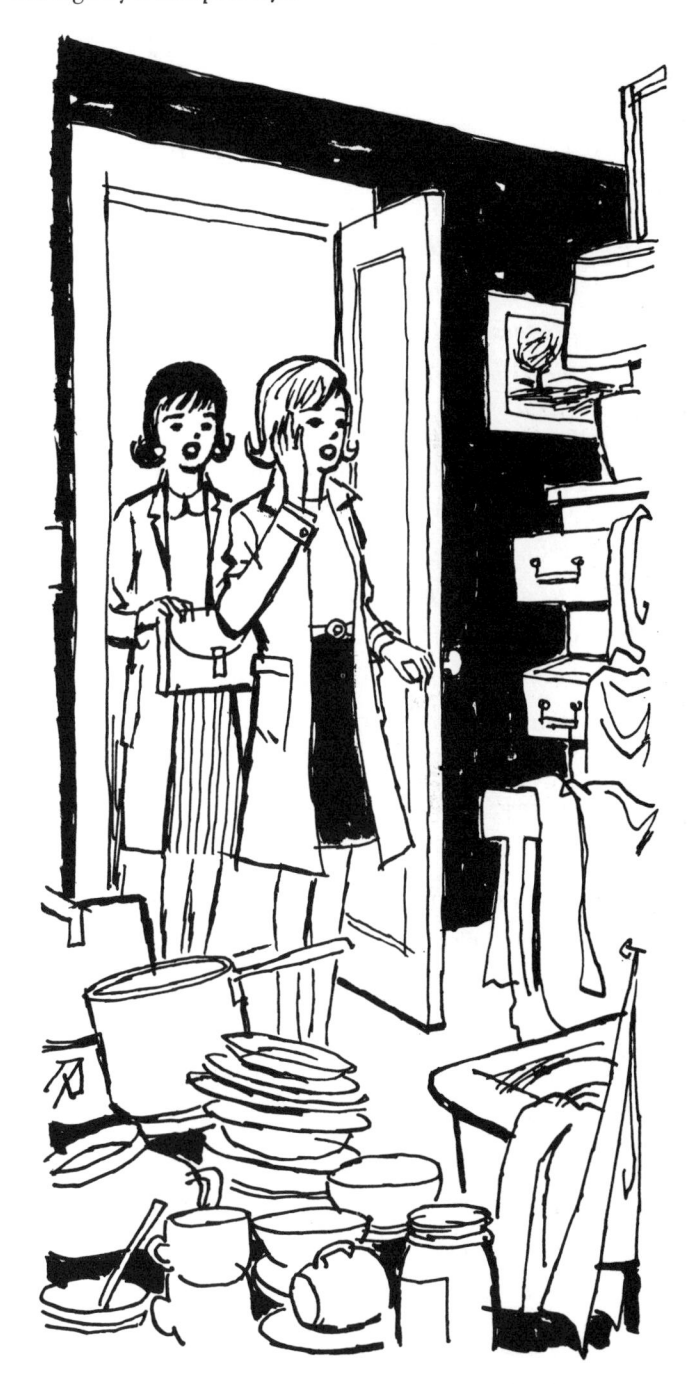

14   a few points to round off the whole

1 *In what you have read are embodied my counsels of perfection. The ideas and routines in the supplement that follows are intended to help you acquire those professional touches that can make all the difference.*

2 *Don't be discouraged if some days you feel you are making no progress in the art of living. Spend a few moments each day building up a picture of what you are aiming at in life. This will help to give you a sense of purpose and direction and to shed many unimportant things which you may have allowed to waste time, money, and energy.*

3 *Learn to appreciate beauty wherever and whenever you find it. Look for it in nature, in art, and above all, in people.*

4 *You could be a crashing bore if you behave, self-consciously, a hundred per cent correctly. Once you have trained yourself in the many ways of perfection, then including them in your life should be natural, unconscious, spontaneous and even inspired. It is this touch of inspiration that can give you an enchanting personality all your own.*

5 *There is no need to hurry on this road to inspired living. There is plenty of time— there is in fact your whole life during which, year by year, you can see to it that your beauty, charm and way of life are enriched.*

If I have imbued you with these ideas, then I am indeed well satisfied

Mary Young

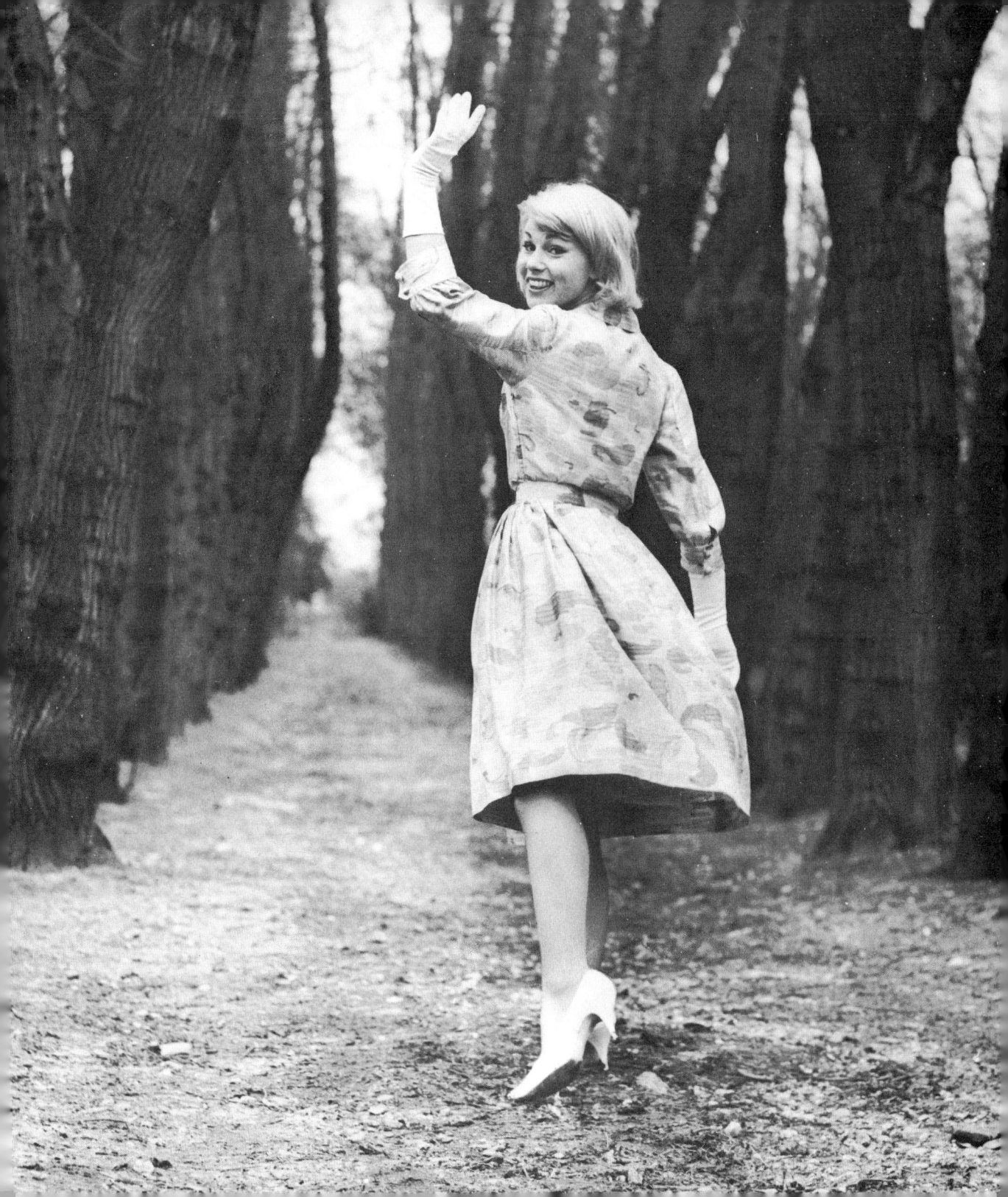

supplement

wearing clothes like a model

gloves

Are they just pulled on or dragged off, somehow, anyhow? The drawing on and the taking off of gloves can be among your most feminine and delightful moments, but *you* must *put* the charm and elegance into it.

Drawing on gloves

1 Draw on each glove by first easing the hand in as far as possible with the palm held upwards.

2 Bring the palm towards the chest as the final easing and smoothing is completed, first at the back of the wrist, and . . .

3 . . . then at the front.

4 Smooth down the fingers into position.

5 Push elbow-length gloves down a little.

Taking off gloves

6 Release each finger a little at the fingertip of the glove, quickly and neatly: one, two, three, four, five.

7 Take a firm, but feminine grip with one hand of the five fingertips of the other glove. Draw off the glove smoothly.

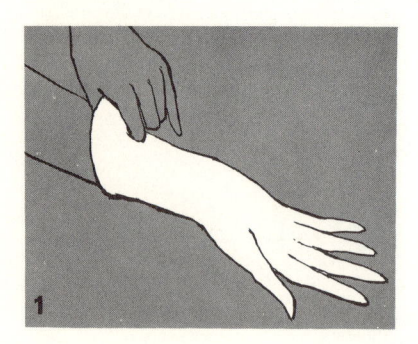

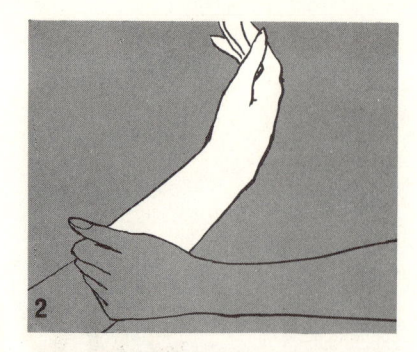

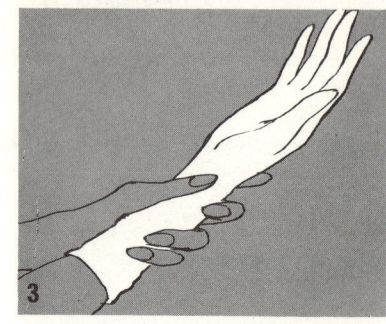

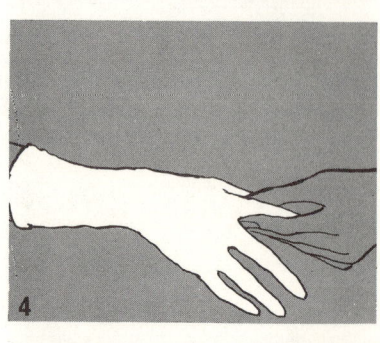

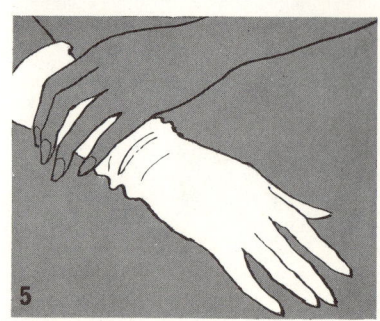

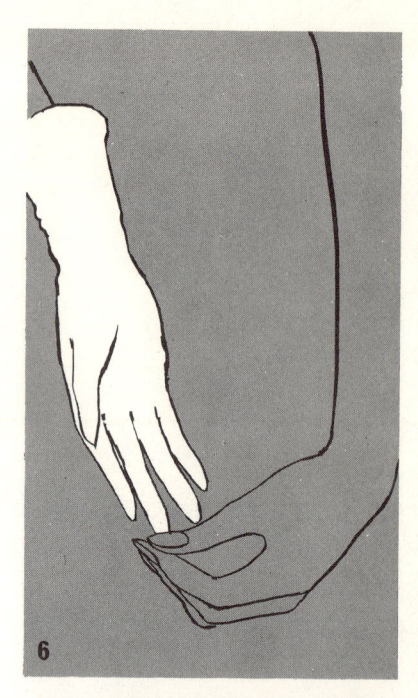

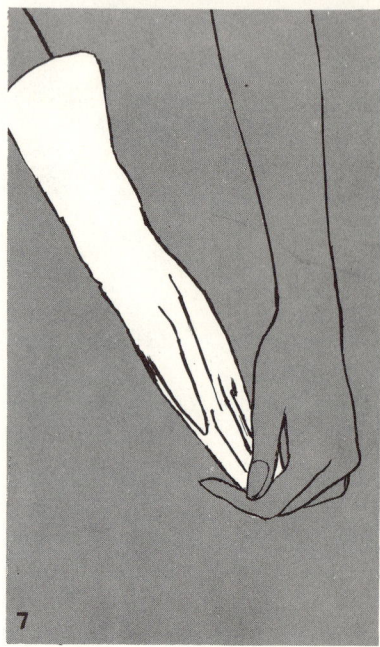

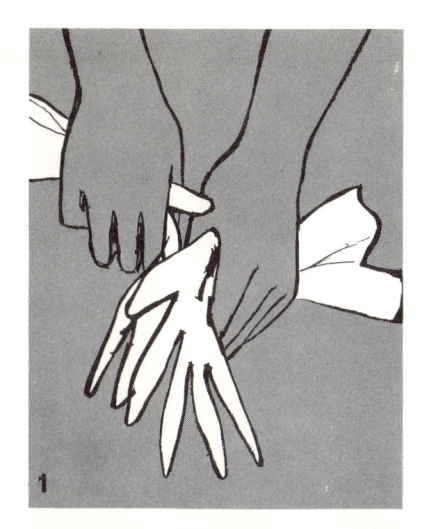

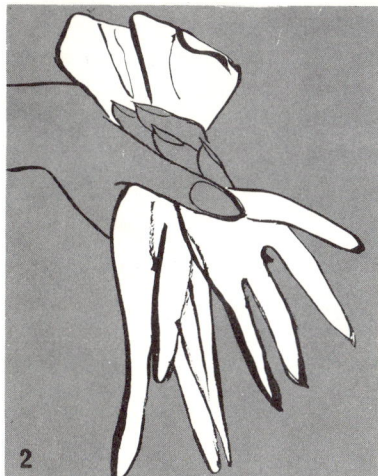

Holding gloves

1 *How not to*—With one glove in each hand.

2 *How not to*—With both gloves in same hand, but with the fingers flying off in all directions.

3 How to do it—With gloves held in the same hand by the fingers, and preferably with the arm held down at full length so that the gloves lie elegantly against the dress.

4 and **5 How to do it**—With gloves and handbag held in the same hand. Try it all out in front of your long glass before leaving home. After a little practice, you will find that the feminine daintiness you are able to put into these little routines can be quite unconscious—quite unlike the Victorian woman of fashion who used obvious artistry to cope with her beautifully tight-fitting gloves of fine kid.

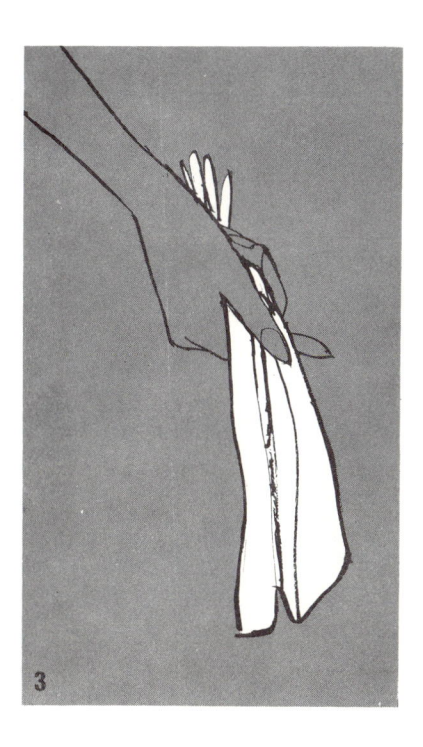

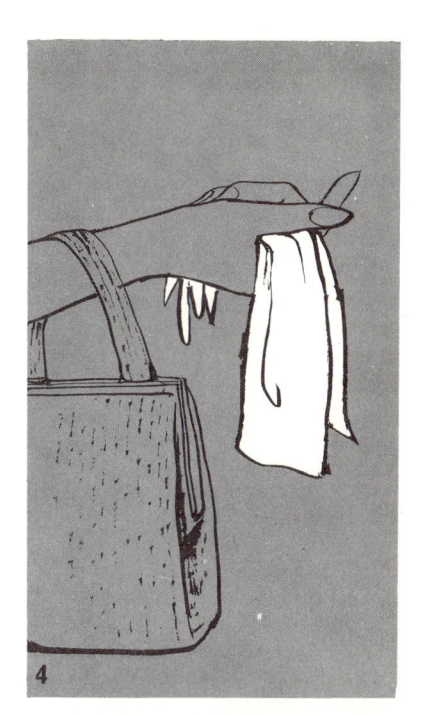

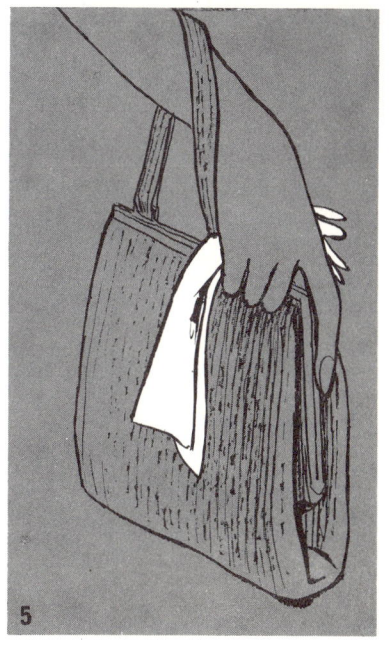

coats

Putting on a coat

1 *How not to.* Flinging on a coat and rushing out without a thought as to whether it is hanging properly.

2 *How to do it.* Left arm into left sleeve, right hand holding left lapel.

3 Use the right hand to draw on the sleeve smoothly.

4 Left hand takes over the position of right hand (in order to prevent the left sleeve slipping out of position). Right hand now released, bends behind the back to get into the right sleeve.

5 Button from the bottom upwards, lifting the material a little to reach the low button (but not stooping to do this—a model must learn not to lose line).

6 Final scrutiny in long mirror for general fit and levelness and for correct positioning of collar and shoulders. Check the fastening buttons for straightness, ease them to the outer edge of the buttonhole. (Sometimes the buttonhole is shaped to a tiny circle at one end, and if so this is where the button should sit.)

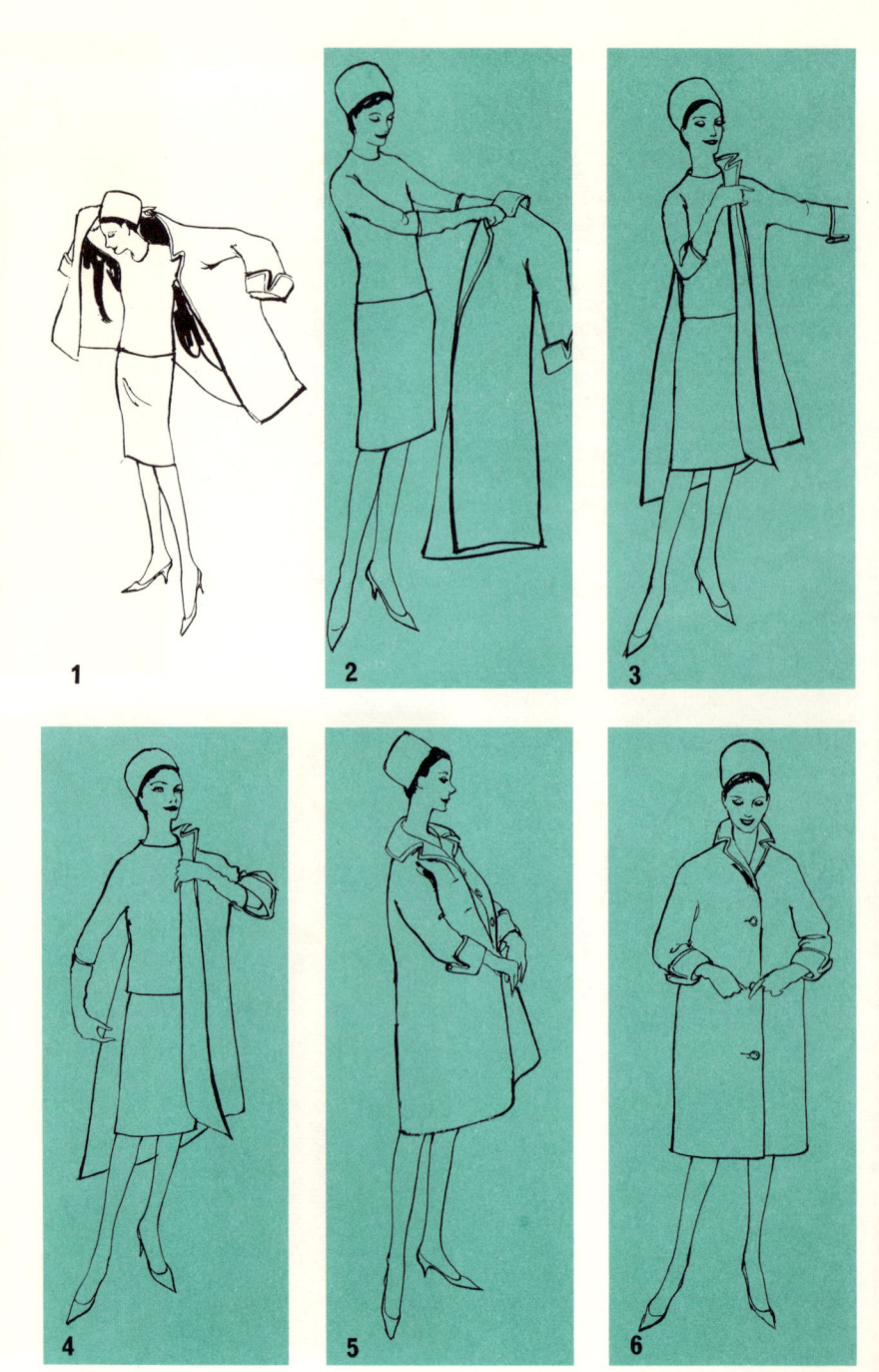

Taking off a coat

1 *How not to.* Peeling out of it any old way—rather in the way a schoolboy would do it.

2 *How to do it.* After unbuttoning from the top downwards, and releasing any other fastenings, bring the hands to a position fairly high up on the lapels and lift the coat just off the shoulders—this can be a particularly elegant moment.

3 Now to the back view. While subtly exerting a little pressure at the top of the arm in order to prevent the coat from slipping, merely take both arms to the back.

4 Draw out the left sleeve with the right hand pulling the cuff.

5 Bring the right arm round to the front, but still holding the cuff (otherwise the left sleeve will be flying in all directions). The left hand, now having taken hold of both cuffs, draws off the right sleeve.

6 Now the coat is off, and you are in complete control of it by having the right hand holding the back of the collar about the middle, the two cuffs being securely held in the left hand.

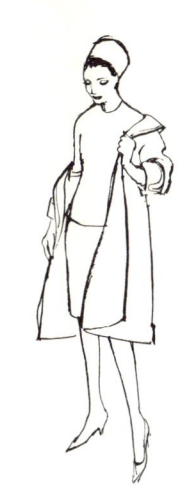

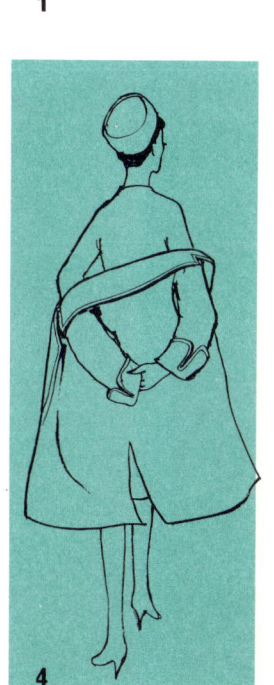

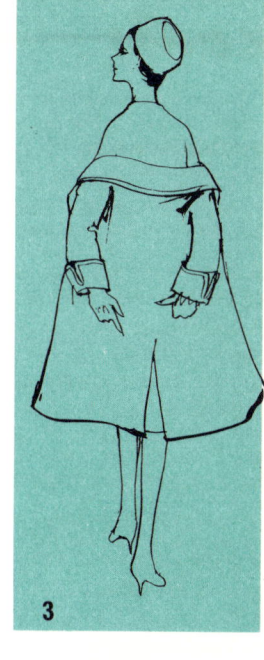

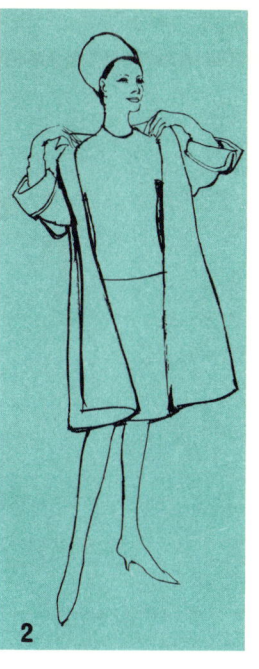

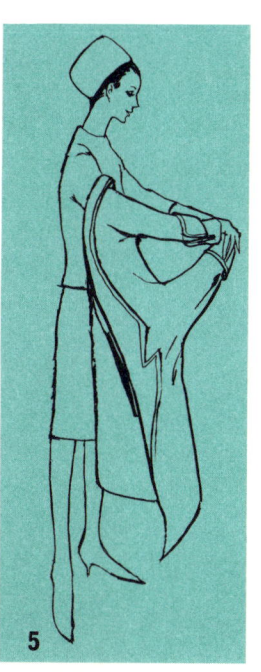

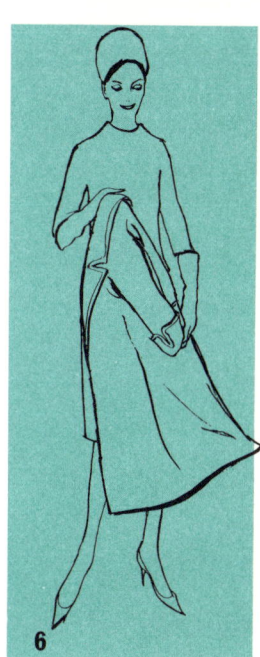

An elegant variation in the routine of taking off a coat

1 At the moment of subtly exerting a little pressure at the top of the arms, allow both sleeves to slide down the arms, catching them at each armhole.

2 Let go with the left hand as the right hand, with a little tossing movement, changes its hold to the middle of the collar—where the back of the neck fits. Bring the coat to the front.

3 This is the moment where the model might luxuriously trail the coat . . . or —with a short coat—just dangle it casually.

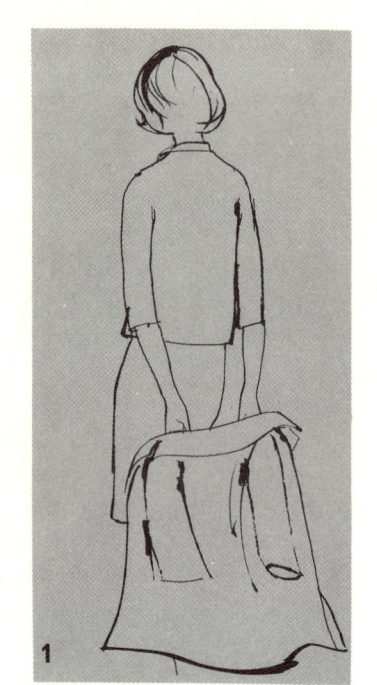

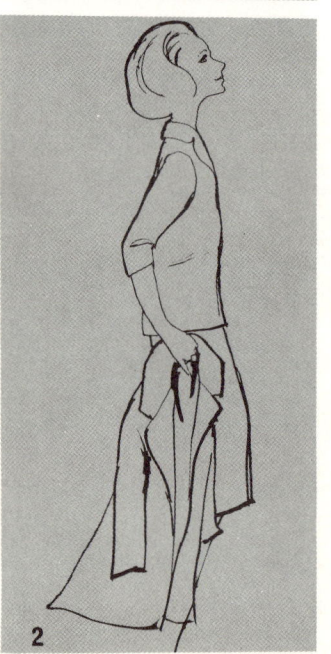

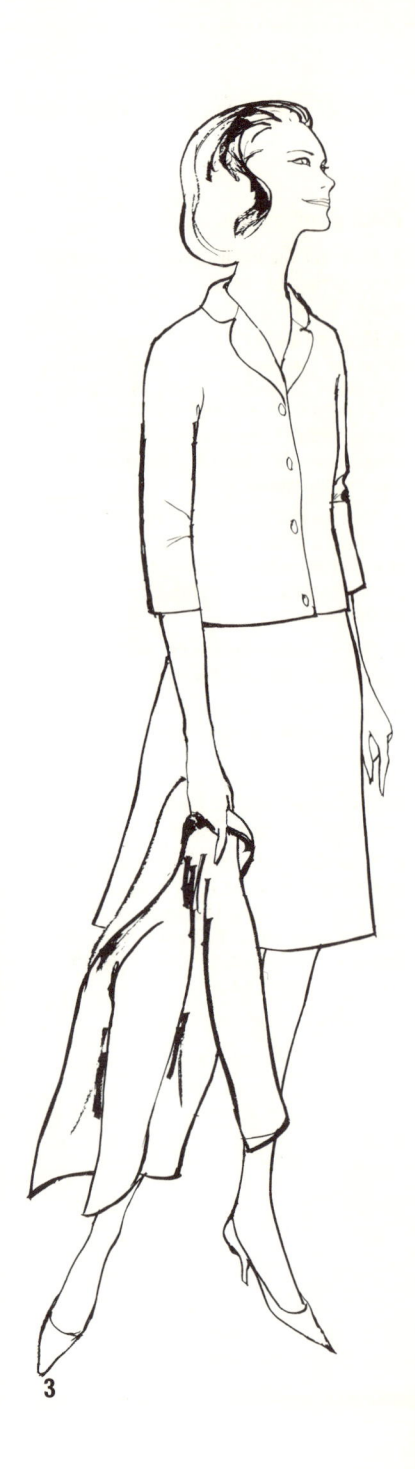

Carrying a coat

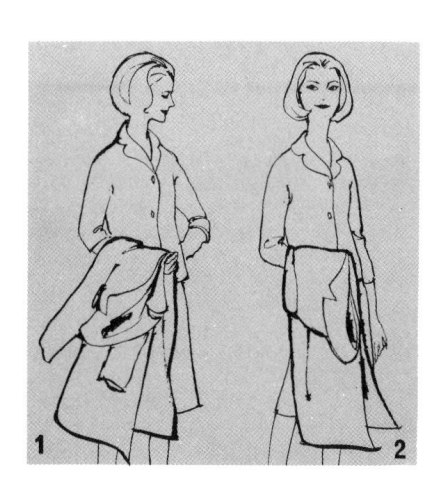

1 *How not to.* With the coat in rather a muddle over one arm, with sleeves untidily dangling.

2 *How not to.* With the coat held right in front on the dress.

3 *How to do it.* In a fifty-fifty position over one arm, with the sleeve just caught up. Hand on hip to hold the coat away from the body is best. The model knows that she *must* hold the coat at her side, and not in front of her where it would hide too much of the garment she is now about to model. You will find that this side position looks better too. Hold the gloves in the other hand, with the arm held downward. Thus you have a satisfying asymmetry.

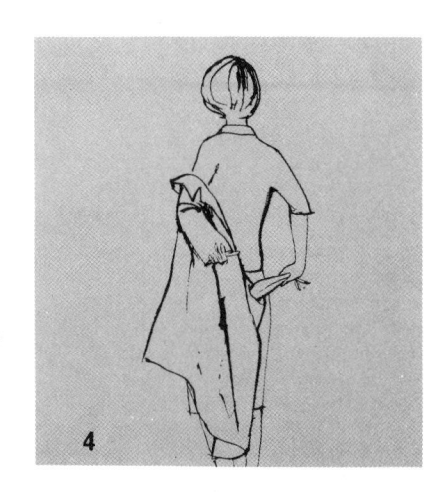

Managing your gloves while taking off a coat

4 *How not to.* Drawing a pair of white gloves out of a sleeve is rather like producing the rabbit from the hat. A model would get a laugh at the wrong moment if she did this.

5 *How to do it.* Keep them on the outside of the coat when the sleeves are being drawn off.

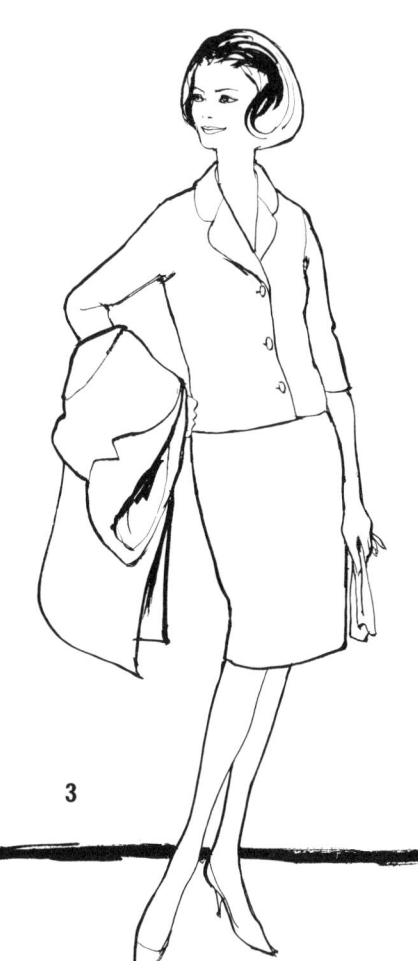

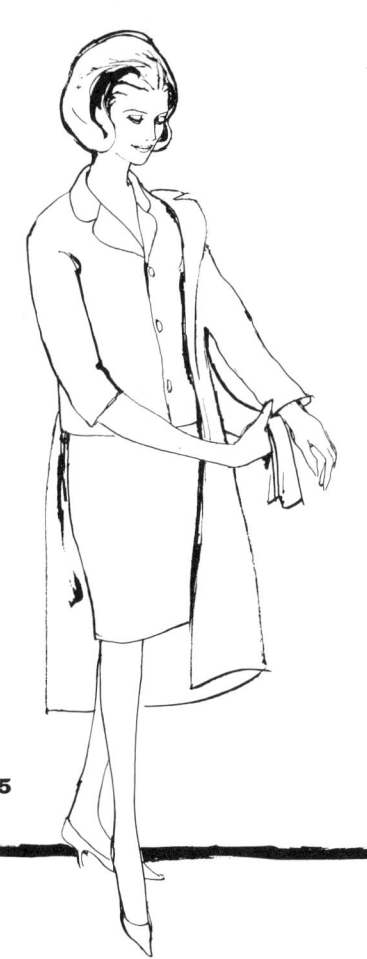

stoles

Have you ever really bothered to try to manage a stole beautifully? A good model can make fascinating play with a stole, particularly if it matches the dress she is wearing, or if it is of some softly flowing material. She will show it in logical sequence, making her entrance suggesting how it might be worn for an arrival.

Then she will move it slowly and beautifully into one position after another to show its possibilities, and finally for her exit she will choose some arrangement with an air, as it might be worn for a departure. Here is a sequence for you to try out.

1 Intriguing Mata Hari style poised lightly over the hair, headsquare manner, but allowing one end (*i.e.*, using about one third of the length) to form a soft face-framing drape under the chin. One hand—it doesn't matter which, try both—must hold the stole in position on the shoulder using, of course, exquisite fingers.

2 Releasing the shoulder hold, with both hands *lift* the stole away from the head and drop it lightly on to the shoulders.

3 *Lift* from the shoulder and allow the stole to come to rest on the upper part of each arm. It crosses the back at about shoulder-blade level.

4 Now ease it to a position whereby it is held in the crook of the half-bent arms, with wrists and hands turned gracefully downwards and inwards so that the fingers can take delicate hold of the stole lower down. After slowly straightening the arms, catch the stole as it falls.

5 Drape the stole over one shoulder and let it fall as floating panels.

6 Lift it away from the shoulder, and place the center under the chin. Then with lovely gestures throw the two ends over the shoulders so that they are flowing down the back. This would be the model's exit picture. She would see to it that by the swift movement of the body and clever use of the hands to fling the ends away at the back, she would disappear with the stole drifting behind her as though it were being blown back by the breeze.

However, the play you can make with a stole depends upon the nature and weight and length of its material, and how it slips over, or sticks to, the dress.

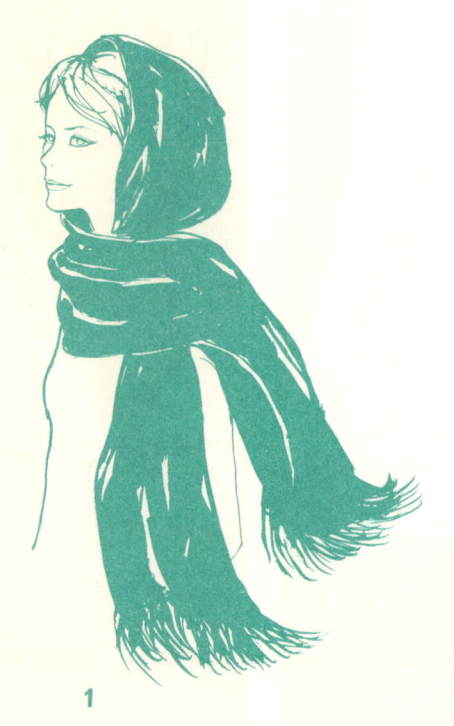

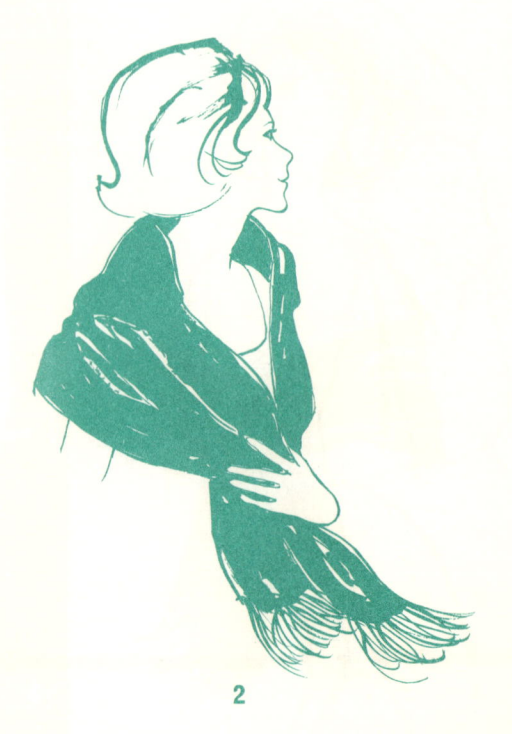

1

2

3

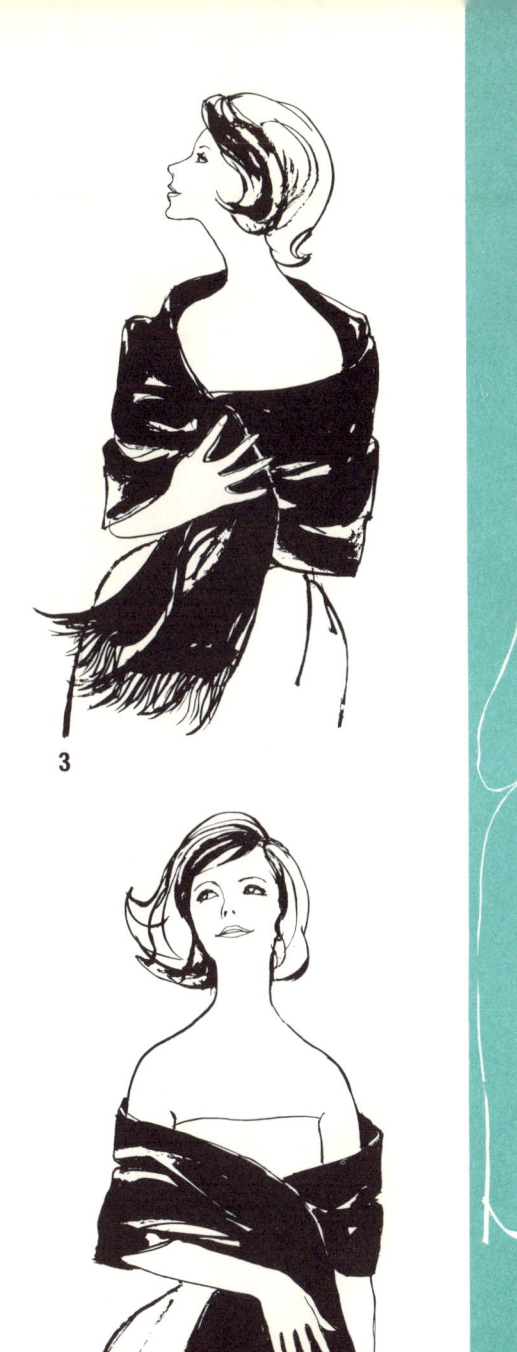

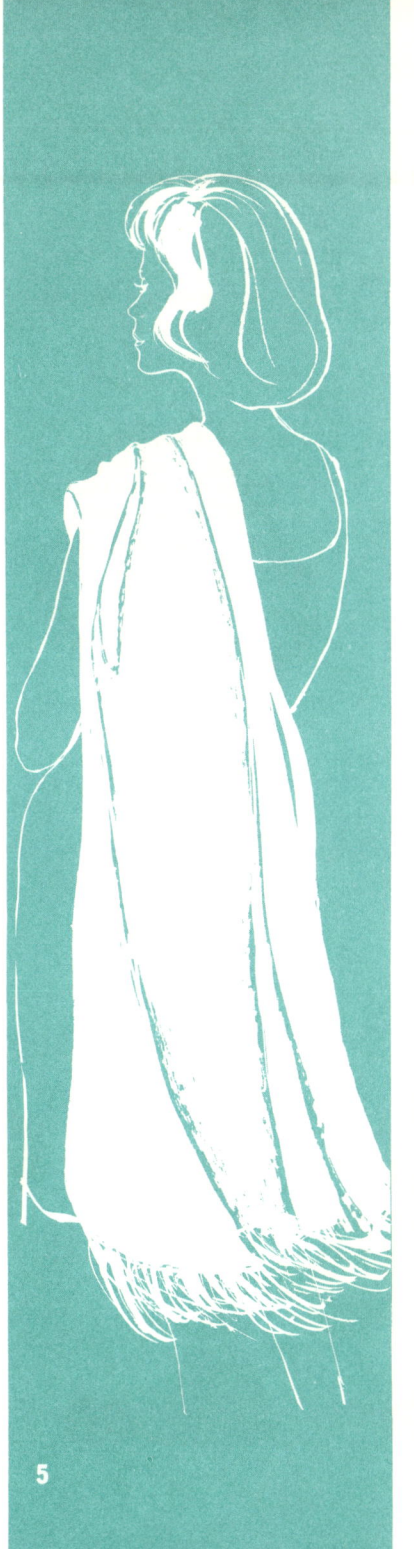

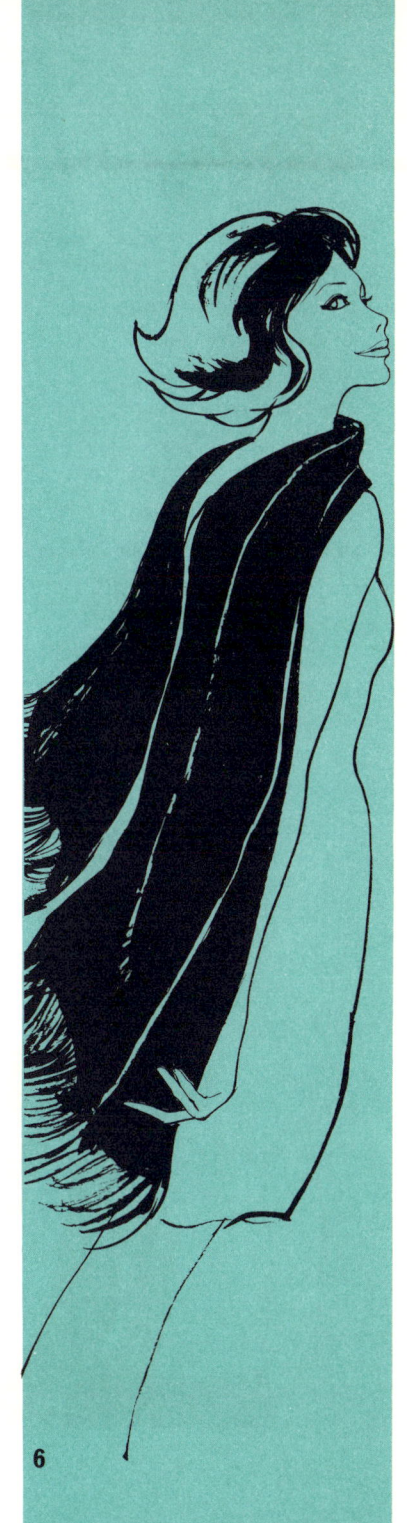

4

5

6

cardigans and jumpers

The model girl is never satisfied until she has tried out all possible variations.

1 Sleeves down to wrist
2 Sleeves pushed up
3 All buttons fastened
4 No buttons fastened
5 Some buttons fastened in the middle
6 Back to front
7 Top button only fastened
8 Bottom button only left unfastened

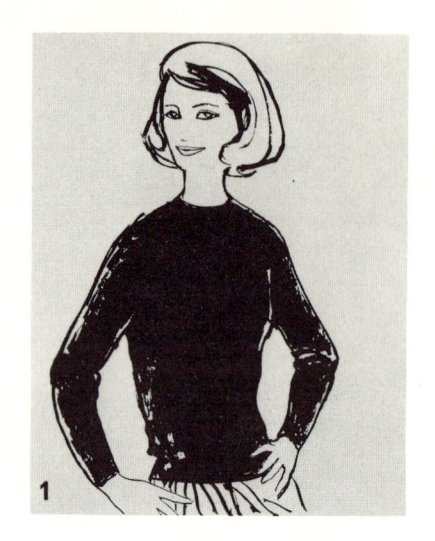

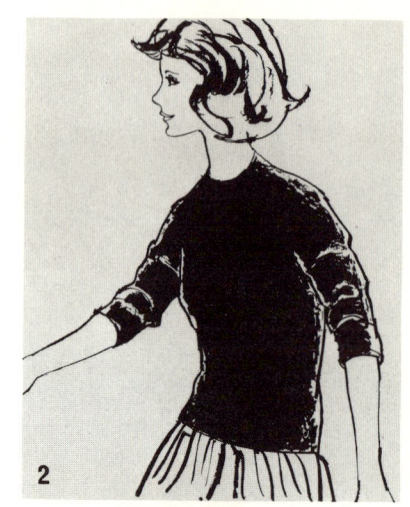

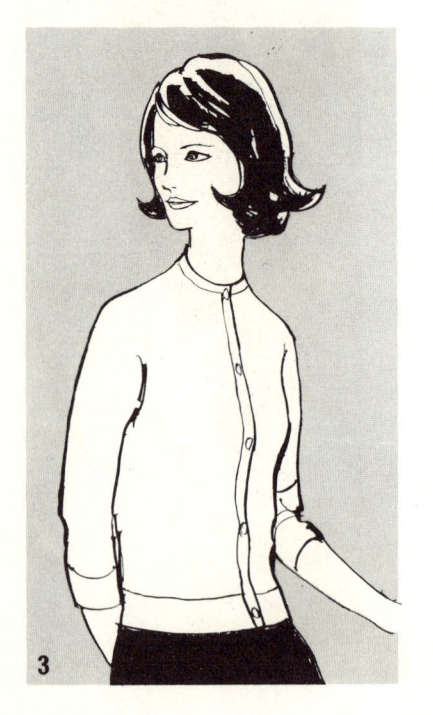

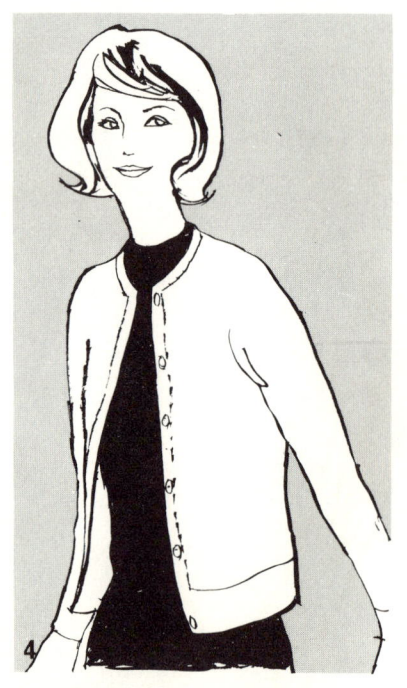

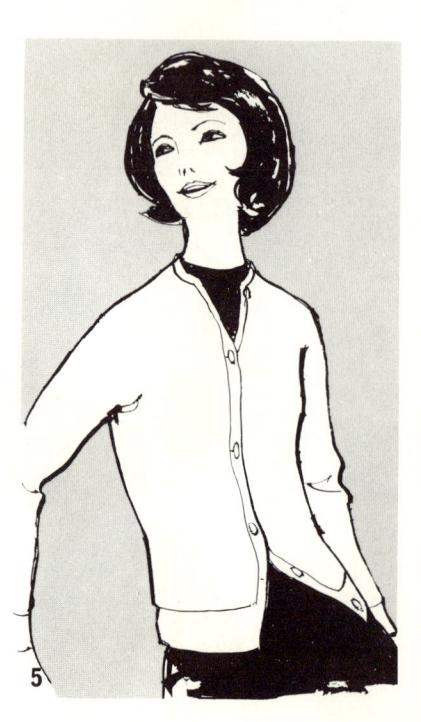

supplement 113

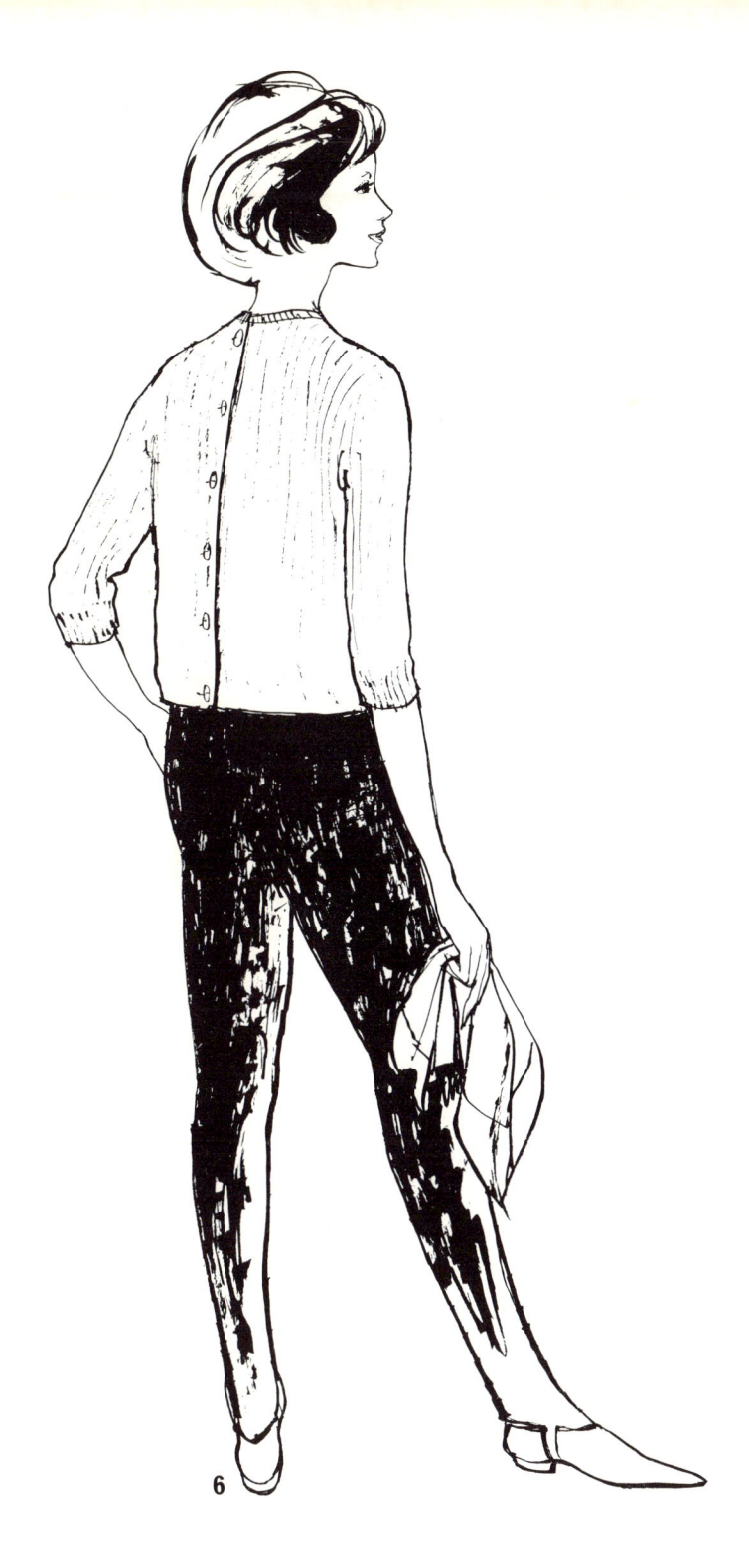

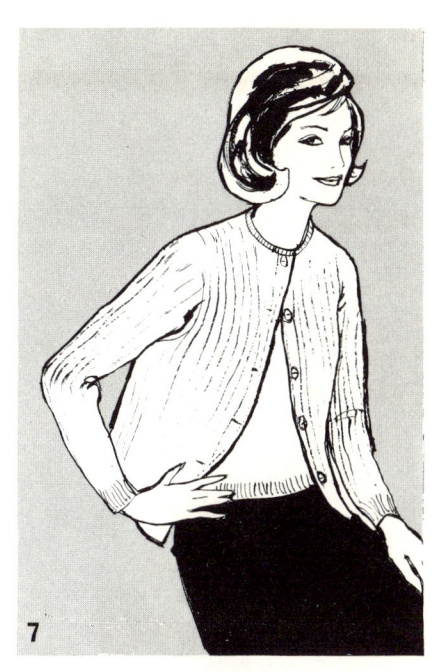

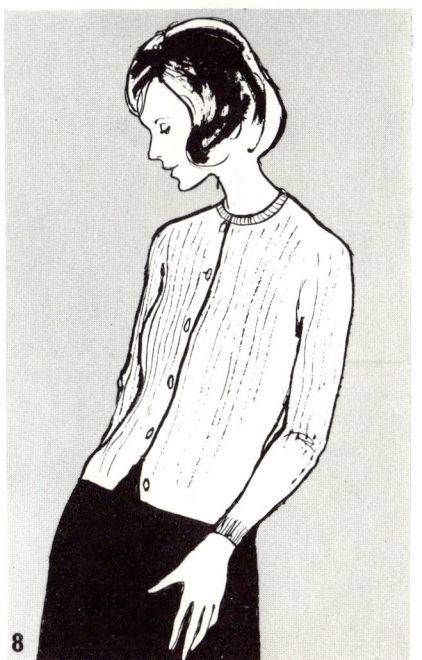

6

7

8

top buttons

Very often suit jackets and blouses with center fastenings and revers look better with the top buttons undone. This must not alter line.

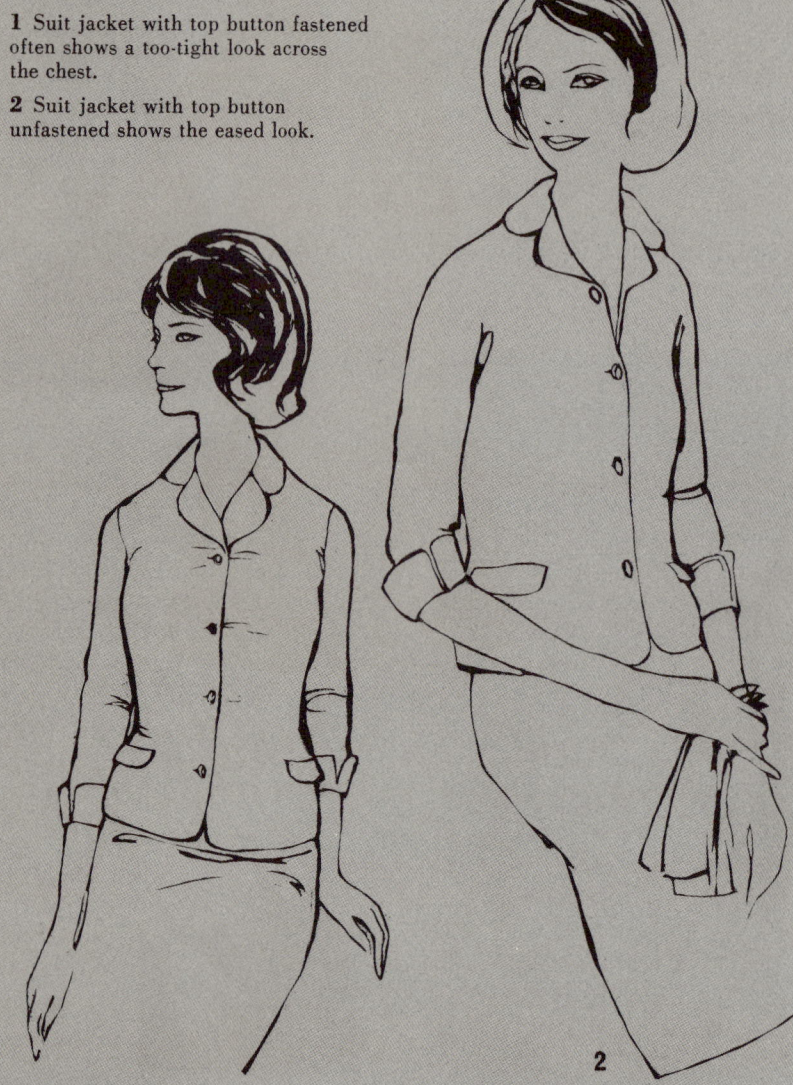

1 Suit jacket with top button fastened often shows a too-tight look across the chest.

2 Suit jacket with top button unfastened shows the eased look.

pushed-up sleeve

No one can quite explain it, but there is something very feminine about the pushed-up sleeve. The model would always try it with dresses and coats.

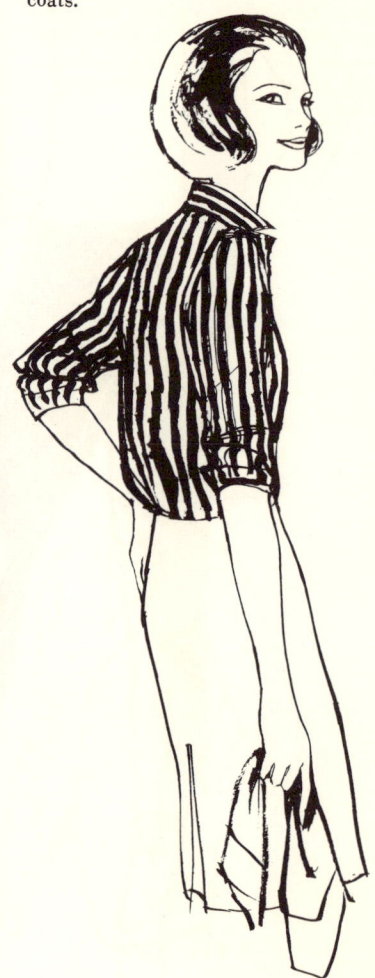

supplement 115

pockets

1 Have your pockets acquired a permanent bulge because you put too many things into them or because you habitually dig your hands to the very bottom?

2 A model only puts hands in pockets very lightly, strictly avoiding any movement that would spoil line. Like every model, once you have assimilated this idea, you will cease to regard pockets as places in which to put things, and the hand lightly poised in pocket becomes merely a self-assured gesture.

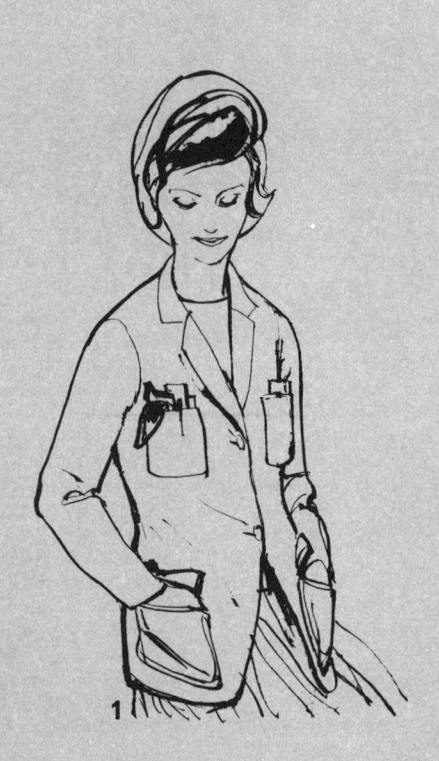

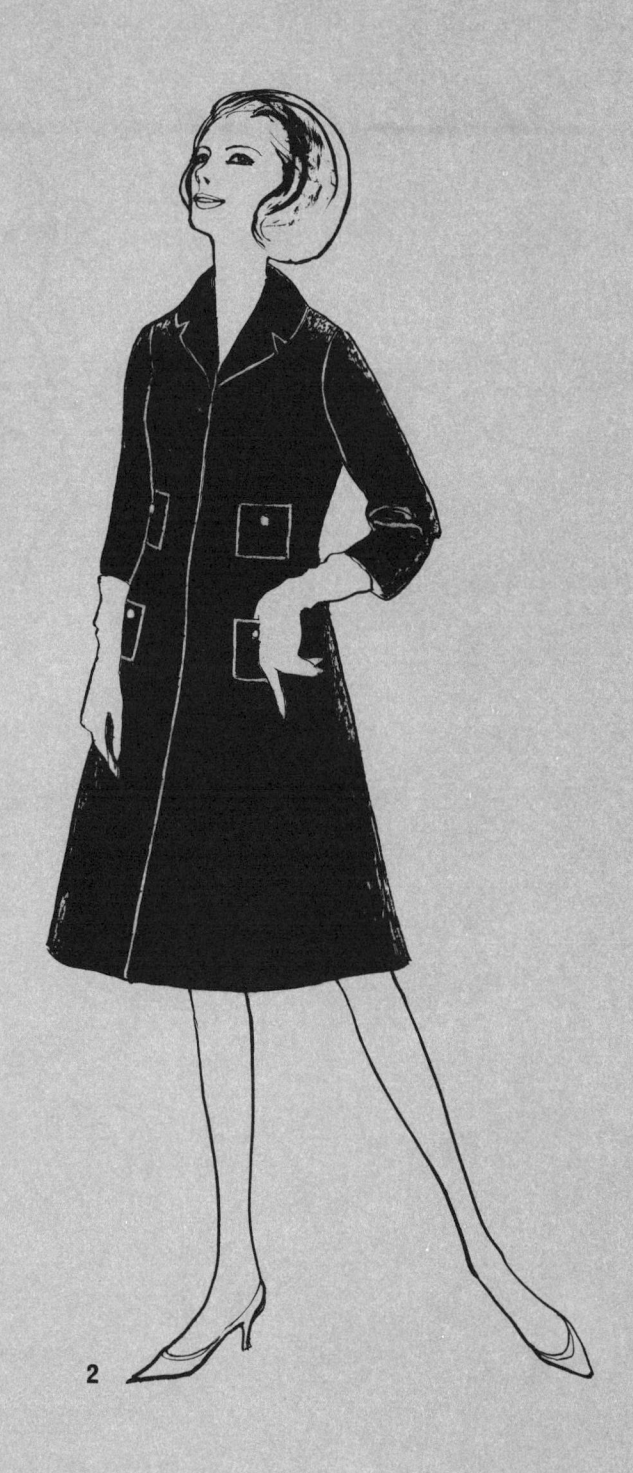

1

2

head squares

1 *How not to wear them.* If you put them on like this, too firmly, flattening out the hair, and tied tightly under the chin, you will probably decide that they just don't suit you.

2 and 3 *How to wear them the model-girl way*—and vastly attractive it can look. The square (at least 36 inches square, and folded over into a triangle) is placed only lightly over the head and is held in position there by two short hat pins, which attach the slightly lifted-up top hair to the scarf and are concealed behind a tiny back fold of the fold of the square. Once you are assured that thus the scarf will stay in position, you can cross the ends lightly under the chin to form a soft frame for the face. The ends, of course, are finally tied at the nape of the neck in a double knot which catches in the angle of the triangle which is falling there.

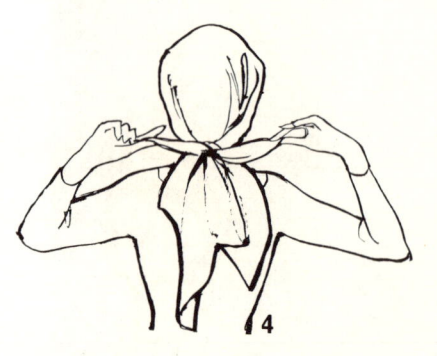

4 How to wear the square the model-girl way over the whole head in order to keep makeup and hair style intact while changing into and out of garments which have to go over the head. The square also, of course, protects the garment from makeup. The technique of putting on for this purpose is similar to the one above except that the square is kept to its full shape, and once it has been placed over the head, the technique for tying is similar, except that the tie is under the chin. One light loose knot is all that is desirable or necessary—the model knows that she must be able to remove the scarf again in a twinkling.

hand bags

1 Does your handbag always lose its line by having too many bulging contents? Do you tuck the bag under one arm and hunch up your shoulders?

2 The model will sometimes carry her bag with her arm down...

3 And sometimes with the handle over the arm...

4 Or, beautifully held in the hand.

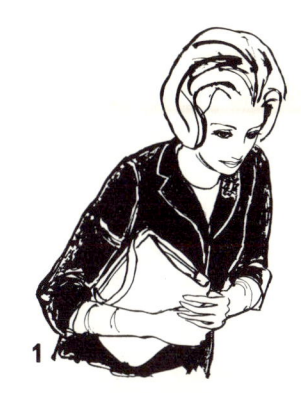

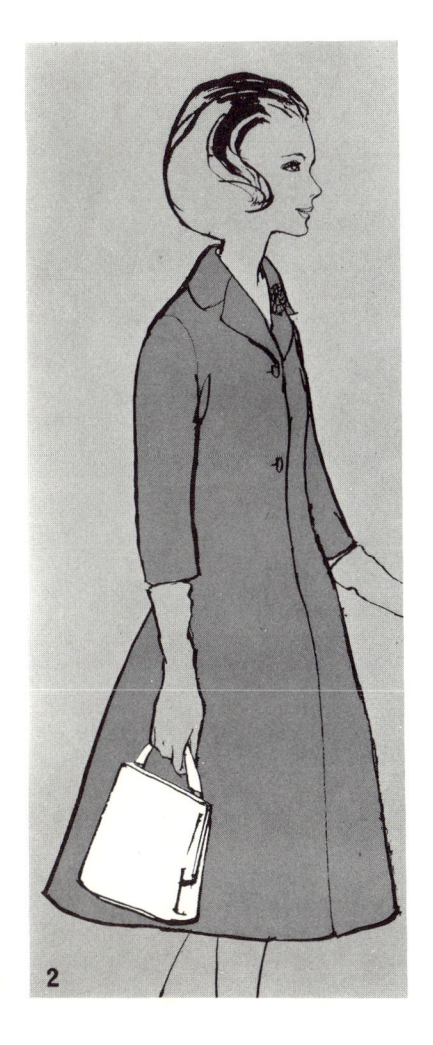

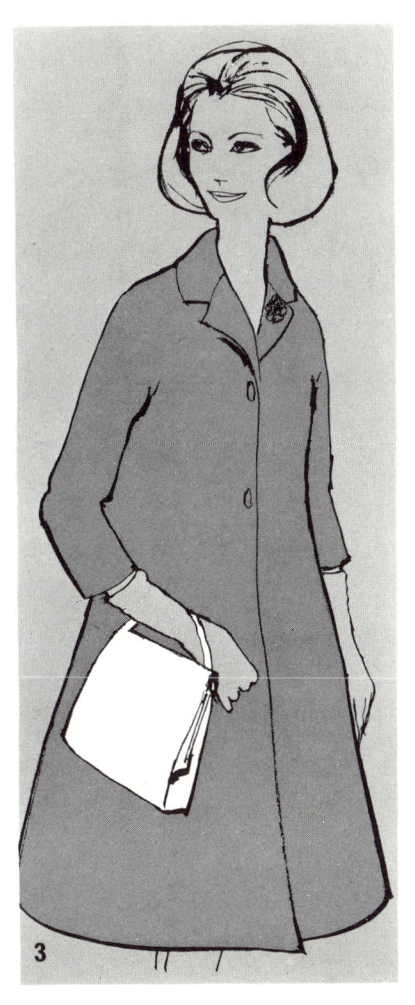

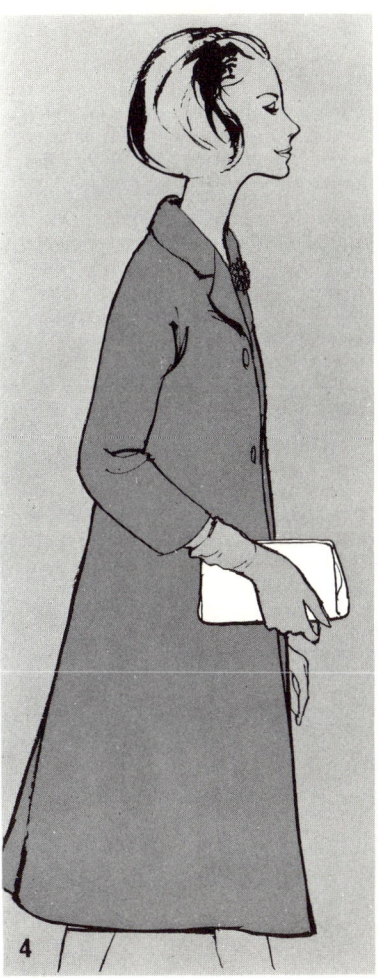

118 IN SEARCH OF CHARM

umbrellas

Have you discovered that it is not so easy to manage a long, slim umbrella with poise and elegance?
Try holding the umbrella handle somewhere in the palm of the hand, with the forefinger stretching down the stem. You will find that this gives you control of the umbrella and prevents any loose, unintended swinging.
Walk with the umbrella in a rhythm of four:

One lift the umbrella and put it down so that it reaches the ground for a second *vertically* at the moment you take step number one with the opposite foot.

Two the umbrella is lifted away from the ground a few inches.

Three by bending the elbow back a little, the umbrella achieves a diagonal lift from the ground. Check that you have maintained the controlling forefinger and that there is a straight diagonal line from the crook of the elbow to the umbrella point. It should be a very steep diagonal and the point should only be a few inches from the ground.

Four prepare for the vertical drop of number one again. Practice this rhythm in an exaggerated way until you've really got hold of it, and then begin to modify the whole thing, allowing the wrist to take over some of the control and developing your own casual style.

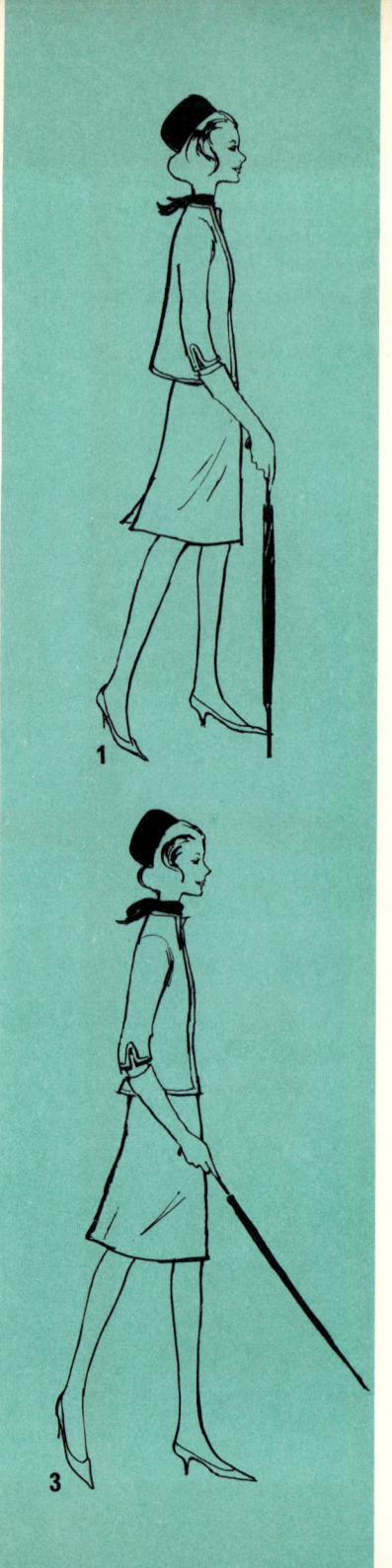

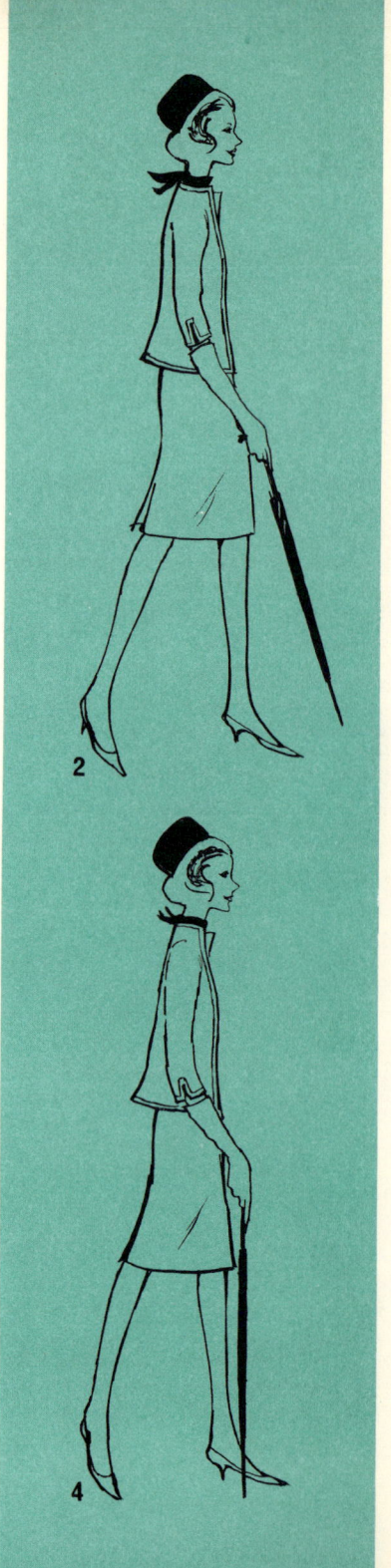

Carrying an umbrella

1 Carrying the umbrella held vertically.

2 Carrying the umbrella held vertically but hooked over the wrist.

3 Carrying the umbrella in a diagonal line under one arm. The diagonal line should be as steep as possible.

4 Carrying the umbrella in the worst possible manner with the line on the horizontal.

5 A model making a very effective stage exit with an umbrella tucked under her arm and her head turned to give a last smile at her audience.

6 A model must be in supreme command of the long, slim umbrella.

As with glamorous hat veils and cigarette holders, unless the rest of the appearance can live up to the poise and elegance suggested, then it is better to leave these things alone. Don't be like this girl.

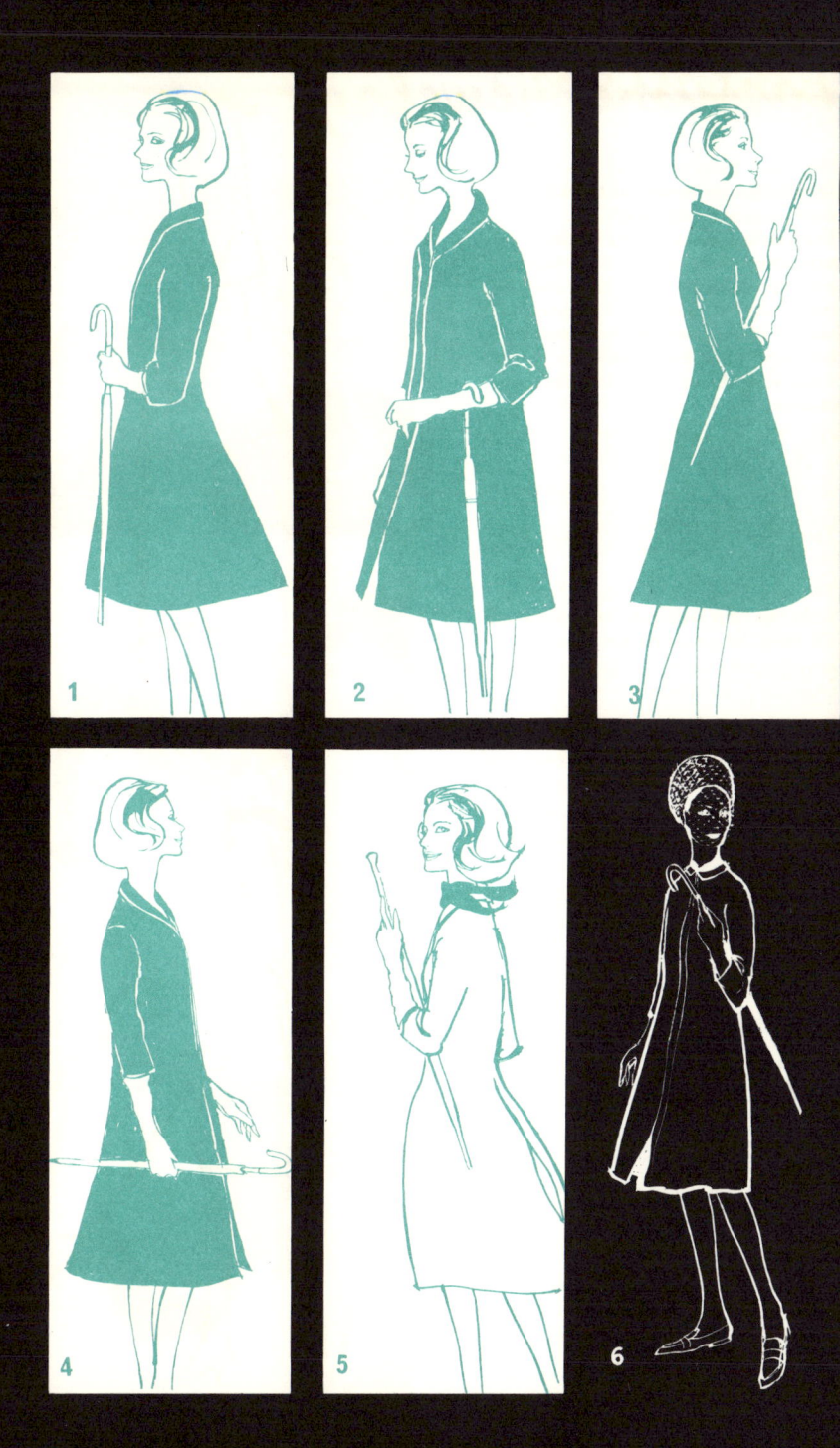

costume jewelry

Do you always wear that little silver chain, or that gold bangle? Each item should be adding that supremely right decorative touch to your appearance—with due regard to texture, color, and line of garments, and no item should be worn just out of habit. A model learns to be up to date, original, and ingenious with her jewelry. Until you have developed your own flair, then experiment with some of the ideas you see in good fashion magazines.

Ropes of necklaces can be worn—around the neck once, twice or three times—or wound around and around the wrist.

Or:

1 Around the neck and looped around a brooch, or into a pocket

2 Bead collar necklace worn as modesty vest

3 Placed effectively in the hair, particularly delightful with an upswept or chignon style

4 Around the neck and knotted to fall either down the front or down the back.

Brooches can be worn at the neck, high up on a lapel (this is a good position for a short girl), low down below the shoulder (this is particularly good for the tall girl), or in the hair.

Or:

5 Low down on a lapel (this is a good position for the tall girl)

6 On a scarf

7 At the waist

8 To accentuate the V of a low back

9 High up on the shoulder (this is particularly good for the short girl)

10 On a hat.

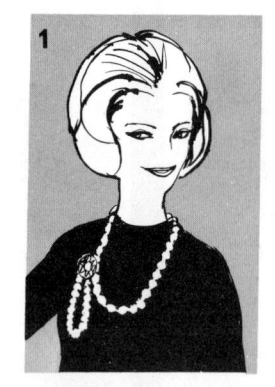

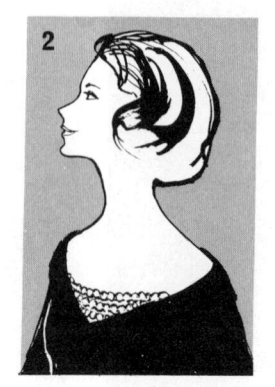

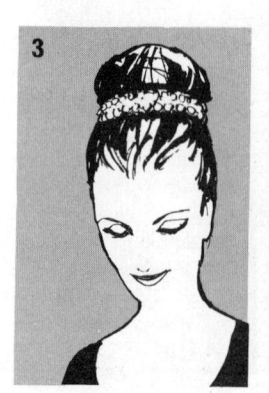

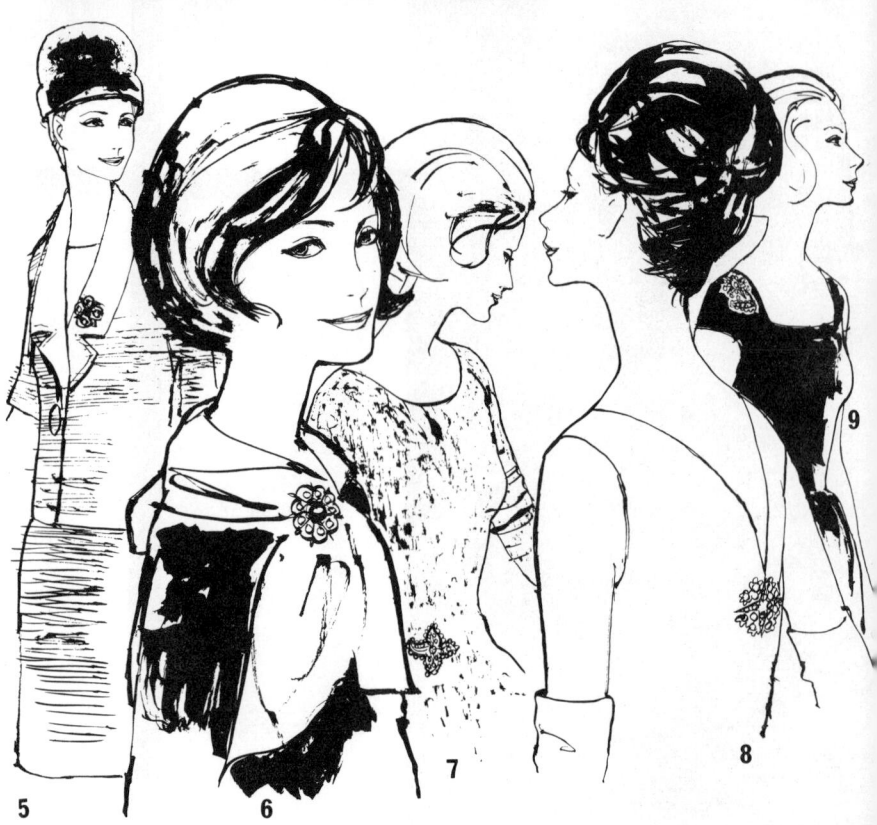

earrings

If other jewelry is worn, then the earrings should be part of the set.

Drop earrings may not suit the broad-jawed face.

Pear-shaped clusters which sit well in line with ear and jawbone can achieve that just-right look.

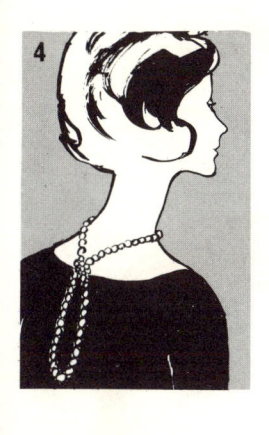

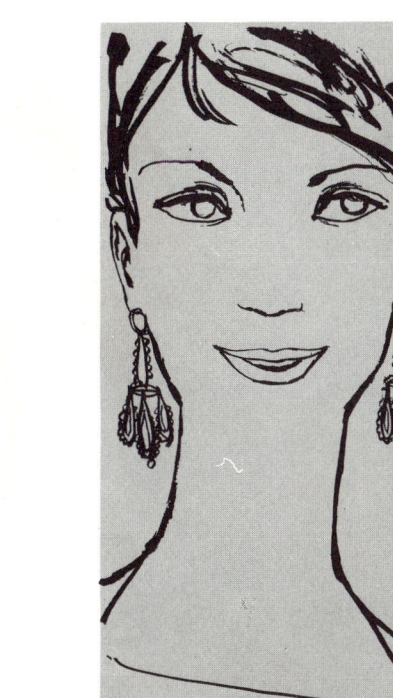

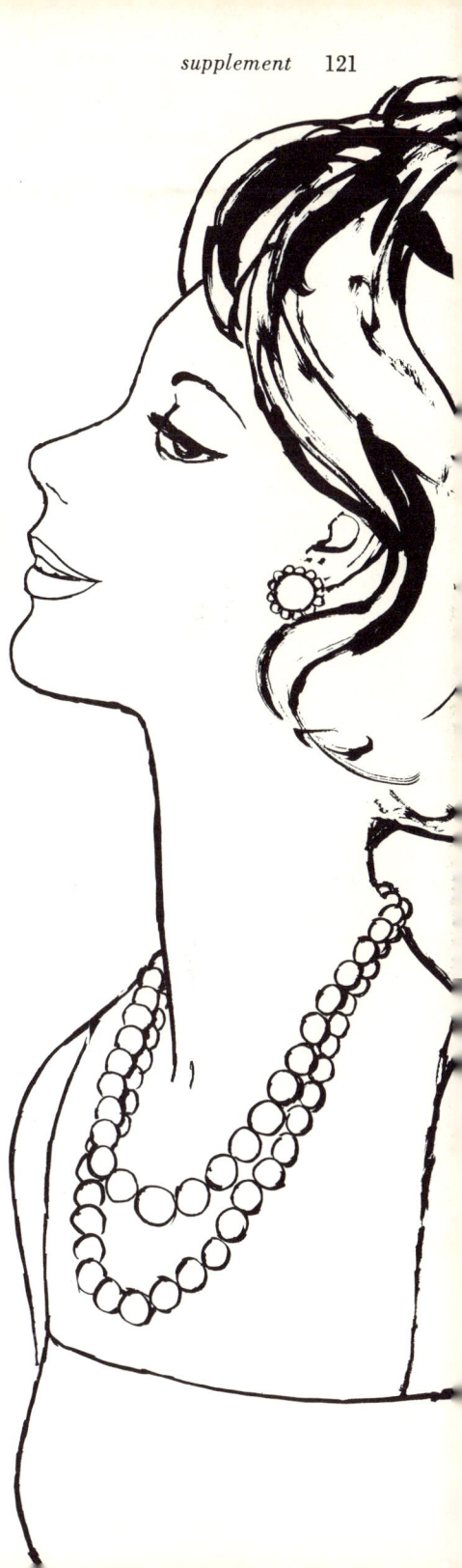

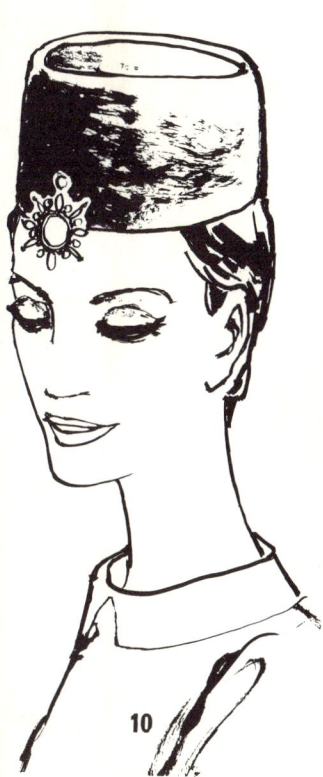

watches

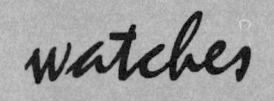

Does your watch look too business-like with your party dress? Consider this, too, in relation to filmy summer dresses and cocktail outfits.

Perhaps change the wrist band to wear with an evening dress. Since watches, engagement rings, and wedding rings are worn most of the time, do choose them with your general taste in jewelry in mind.

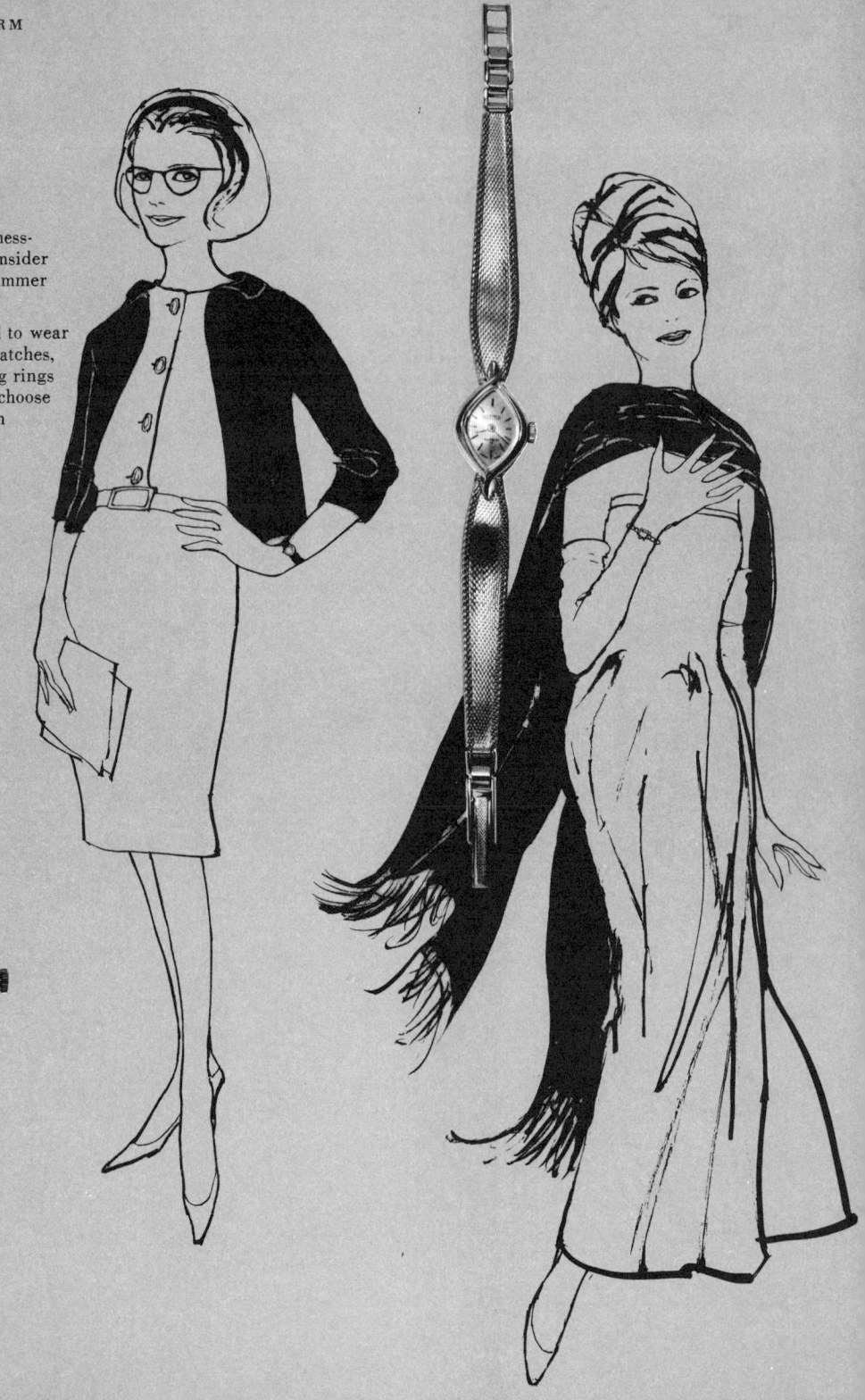